Wasted Wombs

WASTED WOMBS

Navigating Reproductive
Interruptions in
Cameroon

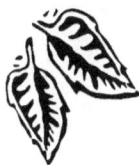

ERICA VAN DER SIJPT

Vanderbilt University Press
Nashville

Library of Congress Cataloging-in-Publication Data
LC control number 2016045189
LC classification number RG632.C17 S55 2017
Dewey class number 618.9320096711—dc23
LC record available at lccn.loc.gov/2016045189

ISBN 978–0-8265–2169–9 (hardcover)
ISBN 978–0-8265–2170–5 (paperback)
ISBN 978–0-8265–2171–2 (ebook)

For Alex and Julia

Contents

Introduction

ON A HOT AND LAZY SUNDAY, toward the end of December 2004, I was informed that a young woman on the other side of Asung had lost her pregnancy.[1] I had already spent three months in this eastern Cameroonian village but had never witnessed an immediate instance of reproductive loss; so far, my anthropological explorations had consisted of mere hypothetical chats about what the local Gbigbil people called "wasted wombs." Now, on this sun-drenched day, the news of Celestine's pregnancy loss rapidly spread through the village and was eagerly told to me as well. Curious yet cautious, I decided to pay Celestine a visit. When I approached the compound people had pointed me to, I found a group of women, sheltering themselves from the sun in a thatch-roofed open hut—some combing and braiding each other's hair, others lying down on the wooden benches, the oldest one preparing a reddish sauce on the smoking fire. The scene was far from exceptional.

After greeting all those present by respectfully offering my wrist to their outstretched hands and answering the usual questions about my health, the amount of sleep I'd had, and the well-being of my family members, I asked if the woman who had lost her pregnancy was there. I was surprised to see one of the lively young women sitting opposite me indicate that it was she. Celestine had a round, glimmering face and deep-set, sparkling eyes. She seemed friendly and willing to talk and immediately invited me to sit with her in her mother's kitchen, "because it is so hot out here and the smoke of the fire might irritate your eyes." Maybe she felt my discomfort in speaking of her "wasted womb" in public. Perhaps it reflected her own uneasiness with the situation.

Alone with me in the kitchen, Celestine offered me a leaf-wrapped cassava stick and, while she nibbled on a stick as well, began to talk about her experience. Sadly, but with a trace of pride, she told me how she had endured the pain all alone, how she had secluded herself behind the huts, and how she had panicked when she suddenly saw a little arm sticking out of her vagina. With the help of a neighboring *mama*, the five-month-old fetus—long since deceased—had finally been expelled and quickly buried. The decomposed corpse of the little baby boy had been a horrible sight. "Maybe it was the heavy work I have been doing in the fields, and I also suffer from jaundice in my belly," she replied when I asked her what could have caused this. Though people had told me that Celestine *herself* had attempted to abort this pregnancy, I did not dare to pose further questions at that moment.

Many lengthy conversations ensued in the months after our initial acquaintance, while we prepared food in that same mud-brick kitchen or worked together in the field that she had carved out of the dense rain forest. Celestine shared her worries about her boyfriend, who was responsible for the pregnancy she had just lost but who seemed unwilling to fulfill his duties toward her and her family. She repeatedly indicated that she was suffering with him, and that she dreaded the prospect of marrying such a "good-for-nothing." For this reason, she admitted, she had initially tried to get rid of the pregnancy. Several failed abortion attempts and a friend's warning about the potential fatal outcome of her interventions, however, had made her decide to keep the pregnancy. After all, she had told herself, her previous baby had also died, and she wanted her only daughter to have at least one little brother.

But then the pregnancy ended nevertheless. Celestine insisted that this loss was not her fault, but due to the illness in her belly that she was now desperately trying to cure. On more than one occasion, she showed me the leaves and bark that older women in the village had given her to "wash her womb." Though her boyfriend had initially financed a few hospital visits and injections "to evacuate the blood," biomedical treatment had to be discontinued when both he and Celestine's mother and siblings—left in poverty after the death of Celestine's father—fell short of money. When I left the village a few months later, Celestine was still under indigenous treatment. Having become one of my best friends over this short period, she cried when I hugged her goodbye. Regretting that she did not have a phone that would allow us to keep in touch, she gave me one of her self-made bracelets and said, "Erica, there are so many things that I still want to tell you. But will you still find me here when you come back? Please take this as a souvenir from me." It is as if she felt we would never see each other again.

One year later, back in the Netherlands, I received a phone call from an informant announcing that my friend Celestine had died. The illness in her belly had persisted and had made her thin and weak. She had gone to her maternal grandmother to seek another treatment, but now the news had arrived in the village that she had passed away. I was sad and confused. But when I called my informant one month later and inquired about Celestine's burial, she told me that the news of Celestine's death had been a false rumor; my friend was now back in the village but was still ill and suffering. The disapproval that I detected in her voice suggested that stories of Celestine's attempts to induce abortion were still circulating, and had made outsiders critical of her suffering.

Expecting to meet my friend when I returned for another round of fieldwork in 2007, I was disappointed to hear that Celestine had eventually died. Her story was recounted many times by women who emphasized the risk of death after induced abortion. Celestine's elder sister Sophie, who became one of my closest informants at this time, nevertheless denied all abortion accusations and told me her sister had fallen victim to witchcraft. She related how a family dispute had induced witches to fill Celestine's womb with mystical water, how the two sisters had secretly visited several indigenous healers together, and how all these *marabouts* had told Celestine that it was already too late and that she would eventually die.[2] Exasperated, Sophie exclaimed, "If she had attempted to abort this pregnancy, the child would have come out immediately, not after five months, totally black and rotten. This was obviously the work of witches and not of Celestine!" Underpinning this witchcraft hypothesis, a maternal cousin confided that it was Celestine's unwillingness to enter marriage that had upset her patrilineal kin. Eager to receive some matrimonial gifts but faced with Celestine's refusal to leave her paternal home, they would "have made her leave" through occult forces—which, in turn, had made Celestine's angry mother move out of the compound and settle among her own relatives. The wife of Celestine's paternal uncle, however, countered such allegations by expressing her strong suspicion that Celestine *herself* had been a witch. Why else would her baby decompose in the uterus and get stuck on its way out? This, she claimed, could only have been the effect of the destructive mystical powers in her belly—which she had probably inherited from her mother, one of the most troublesome co-wives in the extended family.

Clearly, the "wasted womb" and lost life of my friend had caused a big stir in her family and the village. The rumors swirling around Celestine's case remained heated and full of conflicting interpretations until I left the field at the end of 2009. Together, they revealed a complex set of reproductive fears and desires and constituted a powerful social commentary on wifehood and motherhood, gender and kinship, the body and its degeneration, and life and death. Together, they showed that so much more was at play than only the release of that particular five-month-old fetus.[3]

This book is about this "so much more." It examines not only moments of reproductive loss, but also the conditions and configurations that shape these moments and that affect how women give meaning and direction to their experiences. Through this examination, it aims to unravel what is actually at stake when reproduction goes awry, why that is so, and how women maneuver such stakes while leading their reproductive lives. Reproduction is a domain "in which people reconceptualize and reorganize the world in which they live" (Van Hollen 2003: 5). Consequently, instances of reproductive *disruption*—in which stakes may be multiple, contestations complex, and ambivalences ample, as Celestine's story shows—are moments par excellence for understanding the dynamics of this reorientation. How do women and others evaluate, experience, and exploit such circumstances of heightened social ambiguity and bodily precarity? How do such maneuvers affect women's further social lives and their future reproductive trajectories? And what does this tell us more generally about the meanings and management of reproductive insecurities? In providing answers to these questions, this book is ultimately about reproductive uncertainty and potential transformation. It is about wasted wombs and reproductive navigation. Let me turn now to those wasted wombs.

Wasted Wombs: Rethinking Reproductive Loss

Pregnancy loss is a ubiquitous phenomenon. Though rates of loss are acknowledged to vary by locale, it is estimated that, on average, at least 15 percent of all clinically recognized pregnancies end in miscarriage, and that approximately one in fifty fetuses is stillborn.[4] There is a widespread medical understanding that the chances of miscarriage increase with age and that experiencing one pregnancy disruption augments the risk of subsequent losses.[5] Furthermore, women in all times and places have, for any number of reasons, felt the need to terminate their pregnancies. Over a life course that may include multiple pregnancies, women are very likely to experience some form of loss at least once. Celestine and many of her neighbors, friends, and family members in Asung could readily identify with this; as much as 60 percent of the 240 women who had ever been pregnant and who participated in a survey I held in 2007 reported to have experienced at least one "wasted pregnancy" in their lives (see Appendix VI).

But what exactly did these women refer to? "Abum ia digela," they would say. Their pregnancy, their belly, their womb—all potential meanings of the word *abum*—"got wasted."[6] When, how, or why that happened was not specified. Instead, Gbigbil people used this generic term to denote a number of different reproductive events, ranging from early miscarriage all the way to the death of a newborn baby. Even abortions that were induced or, as in Celestine's case, *suspected* to be induced could be referred to in this way. Although there are also other ways of defining and demarcating reproductive endings (which will become clear throughout this book), this all-encompassing and rather fuzzy notion of a "wasted womb" was widespread. It suggests that, sometimes and for some reason, it makes sense for Gbigbil men and women to lump together reproductive events that are viewed as inherently dissimilar in contemporary Western thought. This, in turn, means that any anthropological attempt to understand one form of loss—such as, for instance, Celestine's case—should take into account all the others.

That is exactly what I aim to do in this book. In line with local perceptions, I will take as a starting point all possible forms of disruption that women might encounter during their reproductive trajectories—not only miscarriages, stillbirths, and perinatal and neonatal deaths, but also menstrual regulations and induced abortions. I do so because they are dynamically related to each other, and sometimes even indistinguishable, in people's daily lives and narratives. Furthermore, I believe that it is by looking at different instances of loss, at different moments in time, that we can come to an innovative and comprehensive understanding of the meanings and management of reproductive uncertainties. With such an inclusive approach, I necessarily distance myself from some common classifications of loss. Indeed, the reproductive complexities that I observed in Asung, and that inform my approach, challenge at least two ways in which reproductive incidents are often categorized in Western lay and scientific thinking.

First of all, I take issue with the common distinction between miscarriages and stillbirths. This distinction rests on a time-based understanding of gestation, stressing a gradual development of a fertilized ovum into an embryo, and then into a fetus that is believed to be viable at a specific gestational age.[7] Pregnancy losses can happen in earlier or later phases of this linear process. A miscarriage entails the expulsion of an embryo or developing fetus believed to be unviable, sometime in the beginning of a pregnancy; a stillbirth is the loss of a fetus that would have been able to live outside the womb but dies in utero or immediately following delivery. The separation between these two categories of loss thus depends on the gestational age at which a fetus can be considered viable—a moment that most countries have legally established somewhere between twenty and twenty-eight weeks of gestation.[8] Even if a universally acknowledged demarcation between miscarriages and stillbirths is lacking, there is a persistent effort to distinguish between categories of pregnancy loss on the basis of fixed temporal divisions. Definitions of loss *after* birth are no less time based: neonatal, infant, and child deaths concern the decease of live-born babies within the first twenty-eight days, one year, and five years of life respectively.

That the notion of "wasted wombs" bundles many of these time-based categories of loss suggests that Gbigbil women and men might have different understandings of reproductive processes and losses. This book will disclose what these understandings are, and how they influence the ways in which women give direction to their reproductive life trajectories. Here, I draw on the growing anthropological recognition, spurred by the groundbreaking work of Caroline Bledsoe (2002), that cultural models of reproduction—and by extension, of reproductive loss—are not necessarily informed by a chronological rationale. Physical reproductive processes may be understood in ways that have nothing to do with linear time; categories of pregnancy loss can be distinguished on the basis of other, non-time-based, criteria. The Gbigbil classifications of loss, as well as the flexible ways in which people apply them, illuminate not only the cultural construction, but also the situational use, of local understandings of reproductive endings.

A second distinction I question is the one between unintended and intended losses. Associated with opposite fertility desires and intentions, spontaneous pregnancy losses and induced abortions are generally considered to be dissimilar events, in lay, legal, and academic thinking. Recent work in the anthropology of reproduction—a field that since the 1990s has been explicitly attentive to the ambiguities, contestations, and politics of fertility—surprisingly reflects this dichotomous way of thinking. On the one hand, there are anthropologists who aim to give voice to women who unwillingly fail to fulfill their child wish, such as those who experience infertility or spontaneous pregnancy loss;[9] on the other, there are those who focus on the decision-making processes and controversies around induced abortion.[10] Split by the question of "intentionality," these two literatures address, it seems, two different reproductive domains. Studies that examine the interrelationships between the two are few and far between.[11]

Of course, I do not deny that induced abortions and spontaneous pregnancy losses can have very distinct physical and emotional consequences; indeed they often do. Rather, my argument is that rigid distinctions between predefined categories of "wanted" and "unwanted" pregnancies or subsequent "unintended" and "intended" disruptions do not reflect the potential contradictions, shifts, and ambiguities of reproductive desires and experiences. In Asung, for instance, motherhood is far from always a central aspiration of Gbigbil women. Very often, it competes with alternative projects that women may want to pursue: completing an educational trajectory, finding a paid job, or maintaining profitable sexual affairs with what they call "big fish"—rich urban men who offer them money, consumer goods, and useful connections. In the face of multiple options and constantly changing life aspirations, the desirability of each pregnancy is highly temporal and situational. Reproductive intentions may even shift over the course of a single pregnancy.[12]

The intentionality around reproductive *loss* is, as a consequence, often just as unclear. We only need to remember Celestine's story to appreciate the point: she initially tried to abort her "unwanted" pregnancy and then lost her fetus a few months later, after she had decided to bear the child. Was this loss intended or unintended, after all? That the notion of a "wasted womb" with which people denoted this case leaves unaddressed the question of what, or who, "wasted" the womb only adds to the ambiguity. All that could be pointed at was the bodily event of premature fetal expulsion; the etiology behind this physical disruption was just a matter of guesswork for Asung's fervent gossipers.

It shows that the strict divide between spontaneous and induced abortions is often blurred in practice, and that the question of intentionality is in fact an issue of constant speculation and contestation. Consequently, I do not limit my focus to either one of these categories. Instead, I explore both of them, as well as the ambiguous gray area that lies in between.

By taking an inclusive approach to reproductive loss, then, this book does not categorize events according to externally imposed notions of gestational time or intention. Rather, it casts a wide net to capture a broad range of reproductive situations, interpretations, and ramifications. In line with this approach, I prefer to speak of "reproductive interruptions" rather than of "losses," "disruptions," or "mishaps." As will become clear throughout this book, the notion of "interruption" resonates better than any of the other terms with Gbigbil conceptions of the general reproductive life course, and of the various hurdles that women may encounter along the way. Regardless of the nature and impact of all those hurdles, eventually they represent "interruptions" of what is perceived to be a lifelong reproductive flow that should ultimately lead to the birth of many children.

Next to its empirical significance, the notion of "reproductive interruption" has some ontological advantages. Unlike the terms "loss," "disruption," or "mishap," it does not carry any negative connotations of failure, abnormality, disturbance, and eventfulness. By focusing on "reproductive interruptions," this book also allows space for reproductive happenings that may *not* be experienced in such negative terms. As some anthropologists have pointed out, people's sense of disruption is highly contingent; it depends on their understanding of what is natural, normal, or expected, and those understandings vary over time and situations.[13] Reproductive "interruptions" may at certain moments or in certain situations be considered more or less a disruption, more or less a loss, more or less a pathology, and more or less an event. Not all interruptions are as disruptive as Celestine's; others are less unexpected, less meaningful, more part of daily routine and insecurity, or more easily downplayed as a nonevent.

Reproductive loss is thus reconceptualized: it is transformed from a clearly demarcated and fragmented biological event into a socially constructed and contingent process. As such, it is given local meanings—meanings that are variable, situated in various relationships (with lovers, [potential] husbands and in-laws, female competitors, kin, and gossiping villagers), and subject to contestation and manipulation: in short, meanings that emerge through reproductive practice.

Toward an Understanding of Reproductive Navigation

One of this book's central concerns is to highlight and analyze this reproductive practice. I am interested in the actions and decisions around reproductive interruptions, and in the ways in which these relate to the particular landscape of fertility in which men and women are embedded. Celestine's "wasted womb" was surrounded by various decisions: she tried to get rid of her pregnancy when she discovered her missed period, chose to keep it when these abortion attempts failed, and then responded in a certain way to the unexpected release of her fetus. This all happened while a number of social situations, stakes, and struggles unfolded around her: among many other things, Celestine faced an unstable and disappointing relationship with her partner, serious matrimonial expectations of her paternal kin, financial precarity after the death of her father, fights between her mother and other co-wives in the extended family, and, later on, a continuous flow of gossip about her alleged abortion attempts. A fundamental question in this book is how we can understand the one (i.e., reproductive decision-making and direction-taking) in relation to the other (i.e., the constantly shifting manifestations of various social forces).

I propose to think of this interplay between reproductive action and women's changing lifeworlds in terms of "navigation." My understanding of the notion is inspired by Henrik Vigh's conceptual work on the "social navigation" of youngsters in conflict-ridden Guinea Bissau (2006, 2009). Referring to the nautical origins of the concept, Vigh takes "navigation" to mean "the practice of moving within a moving environment" (2009: 425). When used as a metaphor to illuminate social life, the concept underlines the fact that both people and their social environments are in constant motion, and, more importantly, that these movements continuously feed back on one another. Social life, then, entails "a flexible and adaptive practice constantly attuned to the movement of the environment people's lives are set in" (423). As much as this adaptive practice is actuated by encountered immediacies, it is inspired by people's understanding of the future—their imagination of their social goals and future trajectories in life, as well as their anticipation of the (largely unpredictable) movement and influence of social forces over time. In other words, navigating involves not only acting in the here and now, but also plotting trajectories toward possible futures, and actualizing and adapting those trajectories in the context of continuously shifting social circumstances and horizons.[14]

Though originally developed to account for extremely volatile situations of conflict and war, I consider the notion of "navigation" an appropriate tool for analyzing the decision-making and direction-taking around "wasted wombs" in Cameroon as well. Reproductive interruptions, I argue, present some sort of miniature version of the uncertainty and indeterminacy described by Vigh. They are part of what I—drawing on the work of Jennifer Johnson-Hanks (2006) and others[15]—call "reproductive conjunctures." Reproductive conjunctures are instances in which reproductive contingencies and structural circumstances converge in such a way that they constitute a potential turning point in people's reproductive lives. They arise, for instance, when women unexpectedly miss their period, face a sudden interruption of their pregnancy, fail in their abortion attempts, or lose a baby during or after birth. These reproductive incidents never occur in a vacuum; their happening conjoins with particular manifestations of sociocultural and material structures. Together, the reproductive contingencies and the structural conditions constitute a conjuncture—of shorter or longer duration—in which one's reproductive trajectory is left hanging in the balance. Contrary to other periods in a reproductive life (which may be inherently dynamic in itself), reproductive conjunctures are *critical* durations in which both the present and the imagined future are liable—but not necessarily subject—to transformation.

Of course, there are many such critical junctures in women's reproductive lives, and they are not always related to fertility interruptions (though every reproductive interruption *is* part of a conjuncture). Even one single pregnancy can contain several reproductive conjunctures. Celestine's pregnancy, for example, was marked by two distinct periods of extreme uncertainty and potential change: the first one occurred when Celestine discovered that she had conceived with a "good-for-nothing" whom she might end up having to marry; the second was triggered by the sudden interruption of this pregnancy a few months later. Both conjunctures turned Celestine's life upside down. Both changed her plans for the future. Both implied a twist of fate. While I acknowledge that women's reproductive trajectories are in fact strings of various potential turning points, in this book I will zoom in on those conjunctures that arise around instances of reproductive interruption.

Owing to their inherently contingent, unpredictable, and indeterminate character, the conjunctures around interrupted fertility demand what we might call "reproductive navigation": the pragmatic directing of one's reproductive life through uncertain and constantly changing circumstances. Navigating such reproductive conjunctures means maneuvering through the possibilities and constraints posed by the social and material configurations at play. It also means reconsidering one's reproductive aspirations and future imaginations in light of those configurations, and in light of the horizons—the imaginable potential futures (cf. Johnson-Hanks 2006)—that may appear as reachable and desirable. Depending on the trajectory eventually explored, reproductive conjunctures can become turning points that imply a serious change of direction in people's reproductive lives. Not every reproductive conjuncture necessarily generates major shifts, however. Some are truly transformative; others simply end with a restoration of the status quo ante. Retrospectively, the reproductive interruptions that constituted their core can be seen as life-changing events, or just downplayed as featureless nonevents.[16] Either way, once a potential trajectory actualizes itself and brings along a stable imagination of one's future—whether or not it coincides with earlier ideas about one's future trajectory—the reproductive conjuncture has passed. Others may follow in the uncertain future that lies ahead.

In synthesis with a focus on reproductive conjunctures, my approach to "navigation" differs both in scope and substance from the one proposed by Henrik Vigh (2006, 2009). My "reproductive navigation" is Vigh's "social navigation" writ small, if you will—confined to particular hurdles in one domain of life. To put it in more appropriate metaphorical terms: if the terrains of war described by Vigh could be seen as a huge unruly sea, the reproductive conjunctures that are central to this book are whirlpools on a trajectory that also includes calmer waters. Those whirlpools emerge most often unexpectedly. They can be large or small—steering through them may take a lot of time and effort, or much less. They can change the boat's direction completely, or just sway it back and forth but allow the captain to return to the original sailing route. In the worst case, they can be fatal—involving the loss of one or more lives.[17] But they are always surrounded by calmer (even if still choppy) waters, and it is toward those placid places that the captain will try to direct the vessel. Such still waters can, at any time, turn into whirlpools again. In metaphorical terms, it is those current changes, and the ways in which the captain steers through them, that are of central interest to this book.

Connections, Creativity, and Corporeality

Singling out particular conjunctures that require reproductive navigation—rather than looking at that big unpredictable sea that life as a whole is—has several empirical and analytical advantages. It allows an intimate look at the complex but confined tangles that surround "wasted wombs," and the inventive ways in which women move through them—evaluating shifts in specific social and material circumstances, pragmatically seizing the opportunities offered by the moment, and adjusting their aspirations for the future.[18] Thus, this approach views at close range the aleatory character of reproductive experience and the subjunctive mood—"the mood of doubt, hope, will and potential" (Whyte 2002: 175)—in which women approach the flux of their lives and landscapes. But confining my view to women's navigation of particular conjunctures allows for more than just an in-depth understanding of complexity and contingency. It also helps in discerning how the practices around different reproductive interruptions are socially and materially *patterned*.

Despite their uniqueness, reproductive conjunctures share some common ground. I contend that, regardless of the specific horizons and hindrances they present, *all* reproductive conjunctures lead women to reconsider their previous pathways and their current stakes and ambitions. This is so even if nothing really changes in the end and a "wasted womb" becomes a nonevent. Comparing different reproductive conjunctures, then, allows tracing some general features at play in this process of reconsideration. That is, viewing Celestine's case in relation to the "wasted wombs" of many other women in Asung could reveal some mechanisms of reproductive navigation that are salient within the Gbigbil universe of possibilities. It would help us understand not only *how* Gbigbil women manage reproductive uncertainty, but also *why* they do so *in certain ways*. My aim is to develop such an understanding, and three main questions will guide me in this endeavor.

First of all, I ask how reproductive navigation is structurally intertwined with different, more or less enduring, forms of *sociality* in Asung. Even if the social configurations framing reproductive conjunctures (such as kinship, marital, gender, or intergenerational relations) are highly contingent and continuously in flux, salient social features of one singular conjuncture may resonate with those in other situations. In this book, I explore what exactly these salient features are—that is, which social configurations become relevant when reproduction goes awry—and to what extent they define the reproductive possibilities and constraints around interrupted fertility. How do the webs of interpersonal relations, in which Gbigbil women like Celestine are embedded, shape navigational options during reproductive conjunctures? And are there, perhaps, as Jane Guyer speculated, "specific forms of sociality that *optimize* the occurrence of promising novelties" (2005: 379, emphasis added) at such moments?

Related to this is a set of questions about the social structuration of the imagined zones *beyond* particular conjunctures. The aspirations and imaginations that inspire people's navigation are never simply individual but always derived from larger sociocultural normative frameworks (Appadurai 2004: 67) or schemas (Johnson-Hanks et al. 2011: 4). In Asung, for instance, local ethics of production and reproduction, which portray agricultural abundance and married motherhood as central achievements in women's lives, constitute an important framework inspiring women's goals and actions. But in the face of poverty and consumerism, people also long for futures filled with money, consumer goods, physical beauty, and close connections with urbanites. A powerful narrative of "urban life," presented as the antithesis of rural existence, has come to inform Gbigbil imaginations of the potential lives they could carve out for themselves. Such diverse aspirational frameworks are, however, differently evaluated and appropriated by different people; what may strike one person as a feasible future may be conceived of as an unreachable utopia by another. Navigations differ as a result. In my quest for an understanding of reproductive navigation, I aim to find out how the "capacity to aspire" (Appadurai 2004) is socially structured. That is, I ask how Gbigbil women's positions within the wider social fabric affect which aspirations they *can* have and which ones they cannot, or which horizons and trajectories into the future they *can* explore and which remain unthinkable, when their fertility goes awry.

These (culturally constituted and socially distributed) ambitions can become expressed and enacted in different ways. As the work of Sherry Ortner (2006) has shown, individual projects (i.e., subjective desires and aspirations) may be *overt* and inspire explicit manifestations of power and decision-making, but they may equally be *covert* and less explicitly manifested—instigating, for example, seemingly "passive" endurance or subtle manipulation. Such covert aspirations may underlie the paradoxical situation, also seen in Celestine's case, in which women publicly invoke a notion of passive suffering and social dependence while, in fact, they take their fate in their own hands by means of a secret abortion or other fertility interventions. Covert projects may even be present when women make no explicit decisions at all or seem to comply with dominant structures. Concealed maneuvers like these demonstrate that the plotting and actualization of desired trajectories, though socially circumscribed, involve some degree of individuality, creativity, and, at times, secrecy.

A second set of questions therefore explores patterns in the ways subjective components and individual creativity manifest themselves in Gbigbil women's reproductive navigation. By examining how both overt and covert projects—veiled in what I will call "paradoxical portrayals of powerlessness"—become expressed and enacted during different reproductive conjunctures, I aim to reveal the structural place of *individuality* in Gbigbil society, as well as the constraints and opportunities that reproductive interruptions pose for its manifestation. Ultimately, what interests me is how the social and the individual intersect, clash, or become negotiated in the process of reproductive navigation. This social-individual dialectic has long intrigued numerous scholars investigating the interactions between structure and agency; it is also the topic of a contentious Africanist debate about the extent to which individuality can exist within so-called sociocentric African worldviews and settings.[19] "Wasted wombs" offer a particularly fruitful vantage point from which to scrutinize this dialectic. In the end, nothing is more relational and social than reproduction and its interruption, while nothing is more intimate and private.

Yet, there is something more about reproductive interruptions. Next to being deeply social and inherently individual, they are clearly physical. Whatever the surrounding social structures and individual aspirations, reproduction and its interruption are always intrinsically tied to the body's workings—its capacity or incapacity to conceive a pregnancy and bring it to term. As Celestine's story (or, at least, her own account of it) has shown, the body can be quite capricious: it can refuse to let a fetus go when one attempts to abort it, and it can unexpectedly release a baby when one's aim is to protect it. How do the workings of the material body affect reproductive navigation? And how do such corporeal contingencies relate to the social-individual dialectic? Unlike many other anthropologists who have tried to make sense of reproductive decision-making—whether or not through the lens of conjunctures and navigation—I will take the physicality of reproduction seriously, and view it as yet another potentially complicating factor in the navigational process. I do not, of course, deny that bodies can *also* be inherently social and that bodily praxis is imbued with symbolic meanings.[20] But through an additional focus on materiality, I aim to go beyond mere symbolic and mentalist representations of reproductive decision-making, which tend to overlook the "body basics" on which fertility-related action is founded.

By teasing out the social, individual, and physical complexities around reproductive interruptions, this book puts forward a comprehensive understanding of the meanings and management of reproductive uncertainties in women's lives. It illuminates the process of reconstruction and redirection at play during moments of potential transformation and reveals the ways in which various social connections, creativity, and corporeality contribute to their outcomes.

A Note on Methods

Though I had initially set out to study Gbigbil women's experiences with unintended pregnancy losses, my close involvement in, and ethnographic investigation of, cases like Celestine's gradually destabilized the foundations on which this choice had rested.[21] The more I hung around—in fields, kitchens, thatch-roofed open huts, bedrooms, healers' houses, hospitals, backstreet abortion rooms, markets, and churches—the more I came to question the premises about pregnancy, loss, and pregnancy loss that had informed my initial research questions. My growing proficiency in the Gbigbil language, which allowed me to understand and include relevant local wordings and expressions in my French interactions with those whose wombs were "wasted," only intensified this discomfort.[22] The distinction I had made between early and late loss seemed at odds with local conceptualizations, and there was a constant yet ambiguous connection between intended and unintended losses. I felt I had to broaden my scope to capture the range of reproductive incidents defined as "wasted wombs." And at the same time, I realized that the very processes of defining and meaning giving, as well as the dynamics of direction-taking that derived from it, were intimately tied to the mosaic of the moment in which those incidents occurred. It is these mosaics—the conjunctures—around different forms of reproductive interruption that became my final focus.

As a result, I expanded my group of interlocutors. In addition to those who had experienced a spontaneous pregnancy interruption, I sought to interact with Gbigbil women who had, at some point or another in their lives, passed through ambiguous reproductive moments, such as unexpectedly missed periods and induced abortions, deaths of newborns and older children, or instances of primary or secondary infertility. In practice, this meant that I talked to almost every woman in the village. Yet, there was a relatively small cohort of about twenty-five women with whom I formed the closest relationships and who offered me the most intimate insights into their reproductive lives. Though this book also reports the narratives and impressions of many others—partners, family members, neighbors, friends, doctors, nurses, healers—ultimately, it is this group of women that was most influential in shaping my thinking and writing on reproductive interruption and navigation. My reflections are most often in terms of their experiences.

I studied the reproductive conjunctures in these women's lives both retrospectively and concurrently. Past reproductive happenings, dilemmas, and directions were the central topic of discussion during numerous biographical interviews. Most of these were held during a break or at the end of our working day in women's private fields, somewhere under a tree in the middle of the rain forest. This setting proved to be perfect for sharing intimate knowledge and intersubjective moments: far away from the village, we would not be disturbed by demanding relatives, in-laws, partners, or children, nor would women feel restrained from saying certain things that were not to be overheard by others. The stories thus collected were diverse and highlighted a multitude of reproductive conjunctures—or better said, reconstructions of such conjunctures. Indeed, the sequentiality and intensity of this biographical narrative method exposed the shifting interpretations my informants gave to these past conjunctures, depending both on their prevailing stakes and situations, and on our intersubjective efforts during the various interview moments.[23] Oftentimes, like in the case of Celestine, my discussions with family members, in-laws, and partners about those same happenings added yet another complex repertoire of recountings and recollections.

The volatility of retrospective accounts became particularly evident when I conducted a demographic survey in order to map some reproductive patterns in Asung. Every female villager who was aged twelve or higher and who had been sexually active was interrogated about her family background, her matrimonial situation, and her reproductive history. Eventually, I ended up talking to 290 women. The survey was anthropological in character; conducted only toward the end of the research period, it incorporated local concepts that had proved relevant during earlier fieldwork, and I made sure to explicitly define any potentially ambivalent notion that would appear in the questions. And yet, the answers I received were often confusing. Women would mention stillbirths in the category of "live births" or report neonatal deaths as "wasted pregnancies." Quite often the total number of pregnancies that a woman initially mentioned would not correspond with the sum of "live births" and "wasted pregnancies" indicated at a later stage. Sometimes dead babies had been forgotten; sometimes wasted pregnancies had initially not been counted. Further, several respondents reported a certain number of children to me, while in fact they had been infertile all their lives. Others would denote their "wasted pregnancy" as a spontaneous abortion while outsiders whispered to me that it had been provoked.

Even if such retrospective investigations revealed much about the constant contestations and situational interpretations of reproductive conjunctures, their shortcomings were evident. Generally, people are more likely to remember the conjunctures that became "turning points" in their lives, and they tend to forget about those that *could* have altered their life paths but eventually did not. With hindsight, people may explain the (known) outcome of such "turning points" as the result of conscious decision-making into that direction, and overlook the insecurity, indeterminacy, and contingency that may have characterized the moment. The reverse may also be the case. Redirection at certain moments in people's lives may retrospectively *not* be seen as the consequence of conscious decision-making, but rather, as Cornwall (2007b: 239) has also noted, as "an outcome that needs to be coped with, or a consequence of other choices." In short, the retrospective accounts of my informants offered little insight into the details and dynamics of their reproductive navigation. A better approach, as Jennifer Johnson-Hanks (2006: 198) also suggested when she acknowledged the retrospective bias of her study on "vital conjunctures," would be "to interview women about their reproductive intentions, expectations, and aspirations before they became pregnant, and then to follow them forward through time."

This is exactly what I was able to do when, slowly but surely, women started to share their reproductive experiences with me. They would knock on my door to tell me they missed their period. They involved me in their abortion decisions and practices. They asked me to accompany them to prenatal consultations when pregnant, or to traditional healers when their pregnancy was suspiciously disrupted. They gave birth to their children in my presence. And they invited me to funerals when their babies or children died. Whatever their exact motivations for involving me in their personal affairs—a sense of friendship and trust, a feeling of obligation, the norm of hospitability, pure curiosity, or perhaps the hope for help—women allowed me to follow them through the different reproductive conjunctures that they encountered during the fifteen months of my fieldwork. At such moments, I would ask them about their "projects," desires, and aspirations; I would listen to them when they weighed options and alternatives; and together, we would reevaluate the situation if hopes or horizons had changed. Suddenly, I found myself being part of the very reproductive conjunctures that I was studying.

Of course, this also raised difficulties and dilemmas. In quite radical ways, I came to think about the ethical dimensions of my research activities, and about possible ways to ensure careful ethical practice in the extremely sensitive situations in which I was entangled. The various challenges I faced required an ongoing reflexive enterprise and developed in me an ability to maneuver multiple secrets and to anticipate possible risks and tensions. Indeed, as a confidante, I experienced what it is to live with (reproductive) secrets in a village pervaded by gossip networks and social surveillance. I had to watch my words wherever I went and could not answer freely whenever people curiously inquired how my friends had been doing lately. Involvement in moments of pregnancy interruption was particularly tricky. Aware of the quick eruption and potentially harmful consequences of abortion suspicions, I tried everything to discourage such interpretations. Whenever women actually *did* involve me in their abortion practices, I made sure not to be publicly seen with them.

But safeguarding secrecy was not the only challenge. Being part of reproductive conjunctures also meant becoming entangled in the social tensions that often surround those moments. More than once, I was ignored by the co-wives of my informants, mistrusted by their mothers-in-law, or taken aside by their partners, who asked me to exert influence over their wives in times of reproductive or relational crisis. A close connection to one woman automatically affected my access and allegiance to the others around her. My movement through Asung's social terrains became increasingly complicated as my involvement in individual lives—and the social predicaments and subtle struggles that pervaded them—intensified. Anticipation and adaptation became key elements of my own daily life navigation.

Participating in all sorts of reproductive happenings also came with concerns about the degree to which I *could* and *should* intervene in the lives of those who shared their experiences with me. Faced with conflicting demands for help, moral obligations, ethical standards, and cultural norms, I found this to be a thorny issue. Generally, I tried to keep my interventions to a minimum; and whenever I intervened, I let myself be led by the ethical principles of "doing no harm" and "informed consent." However, these questions turned out to be complicated ones in cases where fetuses were aborted, where the physical well-being of my informants had to be compromised in order to fulfill their wishes, or where not only my informants but also their social relations were implicated in certain fertility-related matters. Given that my own actions and decisions were, as much as those of my informants, part of improvised navigation, I can never be sure whether they were the most appropriate or morally satisfying for all stakeholders involved. Yet, what is certain is that my personal involvement in the reproductive experiences of these Gbigbil women lies underneath much of what I have to say about their lives in this book.[24]

Mapping the Course of the Book

Celestine was never able to tell me her whole story. Many others were and gradually took me on board while sailing the unpredictable waters that their reproductive trajectories proved to be. The narratives and experiences of these women will be central to the chapters that follow. My aim is to situate them in the constantly changing Gbigbil lifeworlds, and, accordingly, to come to an in-depth understanding of the dynamics of reproductive navigation. Hence, the book is divided in two sections: the first sketches the contexts of "wasted wombs"; the second focuses on the actual reproductive conjunctures that are of central interest to this book.

The first two chapters depict the wider environment in which Gbigbil women experience, interpret, and manage their reproductive interruptions. Chapter 1 offers ethnographic descriptions of the social, political, economic, religious, and health "terrains" in Asung, which, together, constitute an unstable and unpredictable landscape that requires daily navigation. I explore how transformations on global, national, and local levels have affected the options and constraints that people encounter in their social lives. The next chapter focuses on the Gbigbil landscape of fertility. I describe women's experiences with being pregnant, giving birth, and becoming a mother, and I discuss the relevant notions of reproductive risk and danger in this setting. The chapter sketches out different perceptions of what a pregnancy is, how and when a "child" is formed, and what modes of surveillance and protection this gestational process requires. It reveals the multiple social sorrows and individual maneuvers that pervade the antenatal phase.

The second part of the book zooms in on the particular reproductive conjunctures around Gbigbil women's "wasted wombs." The various chapters in this section depict the different stakes and situations that may be at play when reproduction goes awry. Aiming to make sense of Gbigbil women's navigation of these complexities, each chapter takes as a starting point the aspirations that women may have while being entangled in particular conjunctural conditions. Chapter 3 explores the meanings and consequences of fertility interruptions that occur when women aim for a future in the rural setting of Asung, in which "ethics of production and reproduction" are dominant markers of status and respect. It describes how reproductive interruptions interfere with women's ambitions to be good farmers, wives, and mothers, and it discusses the options and obstructions women encounter when trying to attain a respectable rural position.

Chapter 4 illustrates how women deal with reproductive interruptions when fertility is *not* their only or primary project, but when they have chosen to pursue projects related to schooling, employment, or rich partners in urban areas instead. It discusses the particular tensions and ambiguities that arise around fertility and its interruptions when women engage in volatile and commoditized affairs with urbanites. This chapter shows how women may turn ambiguous reproductive moments into opportunities for stating their stakes and pursuing their personal projects.

After it has become clear *why* women navigate their reproductive interruptions in certain ways, Chapter 5 illuminates *how* they negotiate and justify their reproductive maneuvers. It does so by describing some discursive mechanisms surrounding different forms of reproductive decision-making. Irrespective of their immediate situations and aspirations for the future, Gbigbil women tactically deploy a shared narrative of suffering, fate, and powerlessness that paradoxically creates room for maneuvering and manipulation. This chapter paves the way for a final discussion about reproductive navigation.

Returning to the three main questions raised above (regarding connectedness, creativity, and corporeality), the Conclusion points out how the reproductive navigation of Gbigbil women is affected by different social configurations, asserted through individual tactics, and possibly altered by bodily states. I also discuss how the encompassing framework of reproductive navigation that I develop in this book furthers our empirical and theoretical understanding of reproductive health behavior, in Cameroon as in many other parts of this world.

Terrains in
Transformation

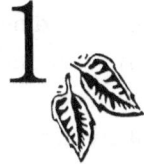

JUST A FEW DAYS AFTER MY FIRST ARRIVAL in Cameroon, I find myself sitting in a rather defective car grumbling about the high speed at which it is being driven through the rain forest. I join Filbert, his older brother, and a priest on their way to their natal village in the East Province, which is also going to be my fieldwork site for the next few months. Having lived and worked in urban areas for years now, the three men seem almost as eager to arrive in Asung as I am. They fill the one-hour trip with animated stories and recommendations about rural life, which seem to gain in liveliness as the volume of the upbeat religious music increases. The noisy joyfulness inside the car contrasts with what I see outside: extended areas of natural beauty and silent forest, with here and there some groups of mud huts. After the sudden fall of the night, only the cooking fires still reveal the presence of human settlements from time to time.

Unexpectedly, in the midst of the darkness and loud music, the three men simultaneously announce that "we have entered the village now." Noticing my surprised look and my searching for cooking fires or other signs of human presence, Filbert laughingly clarifies, "At least this is our terrain. Land is not lacking here. It is our wealth. All you see around us belongs to the Gbigbil people. They have their fields here on which some even sleep or reside." His brother relates how people used to live like that: scattered through the forest. Their current habitation in a village constructed alongside a road is actually the result of governmental pressure, he informs me. The priest comments that, thanks to the abundance of land, people have no problem obeying God's command to "go and multiply themselves" and make this new village grow. Only with a large offspring can they fully occupy and exploit this extended area.

Listening to these lively discussions I notice how, after what seemed a never-ending trip through the vast and dark "terrain," wood fires surround us again and announce to us our arrival in the inhabited part of village. We come to a halt in front of my new home, the local health center. The illuminated brick building stands in shrill contrast to the dark houses that surround it. The light bulb at the entrance illuminates some shabby posters promoting family planning and a lonely goat that has installed itself on the empty benches. The air of desertion that surrounds the place makes room for a vibe of excitement, however, once I enter the patients' ward where I will take residence. The many children of the doctor gather curiously around me, while the baby on his wife's back immediately starts to cry at my sight. Some relatives of sick patients come to greet me. With the help of Filbert, his brother, and the priest, I settle down in the village that I will continue to visit long afterward.

While Filbert's car brought me into the village of Asung, the first part of this book will continue the journey through the local terrains—not only the vast, physical terrain about which my three friends spoke so proudly, but also the metaphorical "terrain" of the village. In its figurative sense, a "terrain" connotes a sociopolitical environment that is "non-transparent and in motion rather than transparent, solid and stable" (Vigh 2006: 12). More than, for example, the notion of "field" (Bourdieu 1977, 1989), a terrain captures the constant shifts of structural organizations that people create, attempt to make sense of, and navigate. This chapter will show that the terrains in which I did research and in which Gbigbil women experience and manage "wasted wombs" are highly unstable and unpredictable. Over time, political fragilities, economic insecurities, deteriorating sanitary conditions, social transformations, and contradictory discourses have come to pervade all domains of life. Such dynamics have affected people's immediate praxis and their imagined worldviews—which, in turn, direct the navigation of the reproductive conjunctures that are central to this book. Mapping the contexts of Gbigbil daily life practice, then, this chapter lays the basis for a deeper understanding of that navigation.

Movements over Time

Asung is a Gbigbil village in the rain forest area of East Cameroon that looks like many other settlements in the region, though it might be a bit larger than surrounding villages; it includes one thousand of the approximately six thousand people belonging to the Gbigbil ethnic group.[1] Their terrain stretches over many square kilometers of green hills, and even the "center" of the village covers almost four kilometers of thatch-roofed mud huts and iron-roofed brick houses, regularly spread along the paved road. Every house is surrounded by one or more kitchens and a hangar (an open, thatch-roofed shed) in which people rest, cook on fire, eat, or discuss. Pigs, chickens, goats, and dogs roam around freely, lie down on the reddish earth, or rapidly disperse when traffic passes on the road—most of the time with a speed that is amazingly high considering its overload. The street is often full of people, too. Children run to and from school with books on their heads or try to sell some *rôti* (humps of bush meat) prepared by their mothers; women walk to and from their fields with huge basins on their heads and with their babies attached to their backs; and men go out for hunting or wait at the roadside with their self-brewed *matango* wine for a rare occasion of transportation toward a nearby market. The air is full of greetings exchanged between people in the hangars and those passing on the street. The atmosphere is peaceful but lively.

While most of contemporary life in Asung seems to revolve around this one paved road, the Gbigbil people were much more itinerant in the past. Until the end of the nineteenth century, inhabitants of this region did not establish themselves for a long time in sedentary settlements but led a semi-nomadic existence in the sparsely populated rain forest. Many of the groups that roamed through the woods would have been driven into the area during various wars with northern Fulani groups from the sixteenth century onward (Billard 1961; Johnson-Hanks 2006; Laburthe-Tolra 1981; Nelson et al. 1974). Processes of movement and migration have been endemic ever since. The Gbigbil people, however, would have been relatively autochthonous to the area (Dugast 1949). While some villagers claimed to have originated in Congo and others tended to locate their roots around the capital of Yaoundé, all agreed that their presence in the southeastern part of Cameroon spanned several centuries.

Throughout this period, the Gbigbil hardly formed a unified group. Social life was built on "segmentary" kinship principles: to become an adult and respected man was to separate oneself from the group, create an autonomous settlement, and become the chief of a new family unit. Power and respect depended on the number of followers (such as family members, wives, children, devotees, or slaves) one could subsequently subject to himself—a "wealth in people" principle that was widespread throughout the region (Copet-Rougier 1985, 1987; Geschiere 1982; Guyer 1984; Johnson-Hanks 2006; Laburthe-Tolra 1981). Movement of the self and of others thus constituted important markers of successful personhood and power.

Yet, hierarchies were never institutionalized in these segmentary societies as they were, for instance, in the centralized *fondoms* in the west of Cameroon (Geschiere 1997a). Men's authority rarely extended beyond the village level and was often contested; family members and other followers could, in the case of conflict or disagreement, decide to go their own way (and create their own group of followers). Those who attempted to gain wider influence on the basis of their personal traits or talents could lose their power as quickly as they gained it—even if they temporarily succeeded in causing upheaval, inducing internal movements, or increasing their group of followers. Domination was thus temporary, fluid, and often based on principles other than kinship. Groups were continuously reconstituted as a result.

As important as the interactions *within* the groups were those *between* lineages. Interclan relationships were characterized by conflicts, wars, raids, pacts, friendships, and alliances. These social dynamics led to what Copet-Rougier (1998) has called a "patchwork pattern of settlement" in which different groups lived and moved alongside each other. Intergroup relations, fed by the constant exchange of slaves and wives, also affected intragroup dynamics. The incorporation of nonrelated outsiders within the group made "belonging" a flexible affair, contingent on sociopolitical circumstances.

In the nineteenth century, this social organization was affected by two major external forces. First, the expansion of the northern Fulbe, whose Islamic jihad directed them southward from 1840 onward, resulted in increased military and trading contact between different clans. As the Fulbe's political dominance hinged on dependence, slave raids, and interethnic hostility, economic and political differentiations became more clearly established in the area. Those controlling the flow of slaves, products, and money were able to acquire a larger number of wives and followers than others. The subsequent development of big polygamous households and of permanent multiethnic agglomerations brought an end to the former mobile lifestyle that had reigned in the region. Meanwhile, the long-standing valuation of social relationships as an important source of power persisted and allowed these settlements to expand (Abega 2007; Billard 1961).

Second, the entry of colonizing forces in the region toward the end of the nineteenth century led, after some initial upheaval and displacement, to even more local stabilization and internal hierarchization. The Germans, and later the French, created fixed villages—an intervention called "regroupement" under the French mandate—that were made accessible and controllable through road connections; they appointed village chiefs who would function as intermediaries between the Europeans and the local people; and they constructed schools, hospitals, and agricultural centers in the communities (Geschiere 1982). All this happened around 1910 in the Gbigbil area, too. Colonial presence and "services" were most perceptible in the Gbigbil village of Ibudim, which therefore started to attract people from surrounding villages.

After a short period in which the annexed region seemed to flourish, the Gbigbil population was drastically reduced, with a yearly rate of –2.5 percent, from 1935 onward. Reasons were the massive rural exodus at the time, as well as the high child mortality and endemic diseases (such as malaria; leprosy; sleeping sickness; and syphilis, gonorrhea, and the resulting infertility) that ravaged the area (Billard 1961; Mengue 1982). Although both colonial regimes attempted to improve this sanitary and demographic situation, the eastern region of Cameroon in which the Gbigbil were located soon came to be represented as underpopulated and underdeveloped.

Although the area is currently still characterized by immense, sparsely populated natural terrains, the Gbigbil population increased again after 1967.[2] This is exactly the year of the massive forced migrations from what are now called the *anciens villages*—or *ilik* in Gbigbil, meaning "what we have left behind"—to the new locations eleven kilometers westward, along a newly constructed road between Bertoua and Bélabo. Because of the low population density in the area and for administrative purposes, the postcolonial Cameroonian government forced separate residential units to merge into bigger agglomerations. In this way, two Gbigbil settlements (called Ibudim and Imanduka) that had previously led separate existences were now forcibly joined into the village I call Asung. The map of the current village construction, drawn by an informant, clearly shows the ordered way in which houses, churches, schools, the *chefferie*, and the health center have been constructed alongside the main road (see Figure 1).

This relocation did not happen without struggle or resistance. Villagers still remember how some were attracted by the promise of "development"

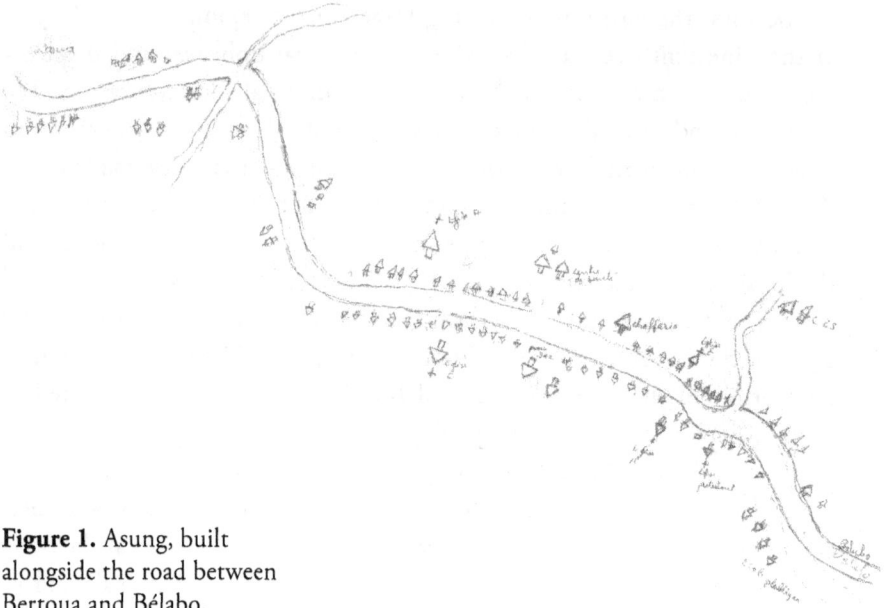

Figure 1. Asung, built alongside the road between Bertoua and Bélabo.

and prosperity at the new location, while others hid on their fields and only gradually started to move their belongings from the old to the new settlements. Old compositions of, and relations between, villages and lineages were drastically changed.[3] Former groups were joined together or torn apart and had to partition the new terrain that surrounded the paved road. This happened mainly on the basis of kinship principles, with different lineages receiving different plots of land. The inevitable frictions and fights that erupted around this division of land made several "brothers" decide to separate from the main group—just like in former times when conflict threatened the harmony of the group—and establish themselves with their families at some distance from the "center" of the village. Some created the hamlet Bitamien (an Ewondo word meaning "let us first try to see") that is presented at the left margins of Figure 1. Others founded the neighborhood of Akepa (named after the river in that area) ten kilometers from Asung.

Moving through Village Terrains

Although ultimately settled, the Gbigbil people in Asung still lead relatively mobile lives. On a daily basis, they move through various heterogeneous "terrains." Paramount is their work in the fields, situated either in the "back-yard" or far away in the bush. Activities in these fields are contingent on the two dry and two wet seasons (*isɔb* and *mbule*) and are strongly gendered. Generally, men give a plot of land to their wives and facilitate the commencement of its exploitation by clearing the field through slash-and-burn methods. Afterward, women rather independently manage the production of corn, cassava, cocoyam, groundnuts, fruits, and vegetables. Much of women's social status in the village depends on the abundance of their agricultural yields, and on the richness of the meals they prepare with it for the children, men, and visitors in the compound. Men may complement these meals with game killed during their long hunting trips, which often involve days and nights of roaming through the forest. Such subsistence activities do, however, not suffice to satisfy other needs or to cover extra expenses. Money is needed for children's education (in Asung's kindergarten, primary school, or secondary school), hospital care, clothing, or bride-price transactions. Also, basic products such as soap, salt, or petrol to light the oil lamps at night need to be paid for—either in one of the three small village shops or at the weekly market where traders from northern Cameroon or Yaoundé offer these provisions at a lower price.

To meet these ends, both men and women engage in some income-generating activities. Many women capitalize on the production of their fields: they try to earn a little money by preparing and selling dishes "on the street" or by trading their surplus products. Some brew wines or whiskeys and sell them in or outside of their homes. Men also go to markets to sell hunted game or self-brewed matango and *mbang mbang* wines. While some older men used to own big cacao or coffee plantations around the old settlements, the considerable wealth and respect they formerly enjoyed has faded away since the devaluation of these products on the global market from the mid-1980s onward.[4] Therefore, young men in particular now create their own fields or work on those of their wives to produce cash crops such as plantains, pineapples, bananas, and palm kernel. The income from these cash crops fluctuates heavily, though, and has become insecure in current times of economic crisis. The despair that inspired the violent riots in Yaoundé in 2008 was clearly felt in Asung as well and has not become any less ever since.[5]

In these days of economic insecurity and political disengagement, where the only reality is just "le quotidien de chacun" (everyone's day-to-day experience), people have created mutual support groups in which they communally strategize and anticipate the future. In Asung, two official Groupements d'Initiatives Communes (GICs), initiated by the nongovernmental organization Plan International, assemble village women under the headings of "We search our lives" (Seying inīng) and "The grain of cucumber" (Sol ngon).[6] Further, many informal neighborhood *associations* unite neighbors for work in the fields, for mutual assistance in case of misfortune, or for weekly *cotisations* in which small amounts of money are saved and distributed.

Though these initiatives might bring alleviation for some, others prefer to escape the insecurities of rural life by "searching for a life" (*chercher la vie*) in urban areas. Only rarely do people from rural areas manage to find a formal job; most end up in the informal sector or petty trade. Those who do succeed, however—like the three men who brought me to the village—end up in ambiguous positions in their natal village: on the one hand, they are respected for their success, their entrance into influential networks, and their role in the village's development; on the other hand, they are vulnerable to witchcraft accusations uttered by kin and nonkin alike. In the light of the egalitarian norms that have long pervaded social life in this region, those who raise their heads above the others are easily suspected of achieving their positions by means of supernatural, antisocial forces.

These and other spiritual beliefs play an important role in Gbigbil daily life. Most of the time, witchcraft stories relate how greedy human beings transform themselves into evil spirits in an invisible world (*mgbɔl*), where they enrich themselves by eating the flesh and sucking the blood of their fellow human beings—who thereupon die in the "visible world." They do this alone or in nightly group gatherings; what counts is that only those who were born with the power of witchcraft (*ivū*) in their bellies can participate and "see" what is happening in that other world.[7] This occult power and the resulting capacity to "see" can, however, also be drawn on for good ends, like combating evil or healing afflictions. Witchcraft is thus an ambiguous power—forceful and often also fearful.

The spiritual terrain is further dominated by Christian churches that have a long history in Asung. The Roman Catholic Church established itself in the region in 1939; the Presbyterian and Adventist Churches did so in 1949 (Mengue 1982). More recently, new congregations such as Mission du Plein Évangile, L'Église Évangélique Luthérienne, l'Église Messianique,

Parole Parlée, and La Vraie Église have also erected their churches in the village. With their active recruitment strategies, they managed to attract considerable groups of followers. Religious life in Asung is thus characterized by diversification and syncretism. As worries about the wrath of God, witchcraft attacks, and ancestor punishments are coexistent and often intertwined, it is not uncommon to see people offer food and drinks to the grave of a dead relative after having gone to the church and while wearing protective amulets against the evil eye of witches.

This variety of beliefs and practices also pervades the domain of health and well-being. For Gbigbil people, healing can happen during a prayer session in the church, with the help of herbal knowledge transmitted by an ancestor in a dream, through the supernatural interventions of a marabout, or after consultation in a hospital. The medical terrain in this area comprises numerous "indigenous" healers and methods, as well as a few biomedical institutions.[8] Asung's health center—my first home in Asung—often represents the first biomedical option for many villagers. Like other state hospitals, though, its services gradually deteriorated since the economic crisis in the 1980s. Electricity and water supplies are scarce, and health personnel and medicines are only intermittently present. The silence I perceived during the night of my arrival in the village can sometimes be found during the daytime as well. Although the only *dokta* (a nurse with some form of medical training) is responsible for the medical care of the inhabitants of Asung and of six other villages—a "health area" that included 6,049 people in 2014—it is not rare to find him unexpectedly absent or suddenly appointed at another health center in the country. In such cases, the clinic can be deserted for days, weeks, or even months on end.[9]

For such reasons, many people prefer to use the sanitary services of the Roman Catholic missionary station that was built in the 1930s in the old settlement of Kamandjom and was later moved toward the paved road at a few kilometers distance from Asung. It is currently led by Italian, Brazilian, and Cameroonian sisters.[10] The medical services it provides are perceived to be better and more continuous than those offered in state institutions. The sisters also organize educative workshops on food preparation and hygiene for pregnant women, young mothers, and people living with HIV/AIDS. Although nowadays patients of all religious backgrounds are accepted and treated in the missionary health station, the care remains strongly guided by Christian principles; family planning advertisements and services are formally absent.[11] For those services, as well as for more complicated medical issues, people mostly resort to hospitals in Bélabo or Bertoua, each of them situated at the end of the road that traverses the village of Asung.

This road, then, not only tied the local population to their sedentary settlements but has also permitted people's constant mobility while they navigate the different domains of life. The schools, churches, shops, and medical establishments that can be found along its sides have also attracted other ethnic groups to Asung. Over time, Muslims from northern Cameroon have come to settle down, initiate commerce, or offer their paid labor force. The arrival and integration of different ethnicities has brought a diversity of languages to Asung; next to the local language of the Gbigbil people—which carries the same name as the ethnic group[12]—almost everybody uses the French language as a lingua franca when communicating with old and new neighbors, when negotiating with foreign traders in local markets, or when traveling to relatives in urban areas. Such diversity and mobility is, however, not only the result of an itinerant history and a dynamic present. It is also inherently linked to complex marital and kinship relationships.

"A Daughter Is to Be Shared":
Marriage Arrangements and Kinship Idioms

The Gbigbil people in Asung are subdivided into nine extended patrilineal families (*metum*, singular *atum*), of which the most prominent is the Bibakung lineage. Members of an atum live together in a spatially demarcated neighborhood, called *quartier* in French or *itounsung*—meaning "small village"—in Gbigbil. These quartiers are inhabited by the male descendants of a common ancestor and their wives, as well as their sons and unmarried daughters.[13] Most of the metum in Asung intermarry, but exogamy is prescribed with regard to the kin groups of both one's father and one's mother. The official rule traces predecessors of both parents into the fourth generation and forbids marriage between all respective descendants. Even if, in practice, this rule seems more complicated (as there are some exceptions on the matrilateral side) and more contested (especially when members of the third or fourth generation have died), its nonadherence is generally believed to result in the death of the married partners or their children.[14] Knowledge of genealogies is therefore deemed indispensable in the search for suitable marriage candidates. "One ngon/mo nye?" (of whom are you a daughter/son?) is the initial inquiry in this respect, followed by the question "niaŋa ane ngon nye?" meaning "of whom is your mother a daughter?"

This importance of genealogical knowledge dates back to earlier, non-sedentary times. Notions of descent would define the interactions between migrating groups who would run into each other in the forest. If they could trace a common ancestor, nobody would be killed; if they perceived themselves to be unrelated, they would treat each other as potential enemies. Relationships between potential enemies could range from actual war to bonds of friendship or even marriage. Because of the rule of exogamy, it was only among those nonrelated groups that conjugal partners were to be chosen; marriage always implied a relationship of dependence between possible foes. The local saying "marriage is war" (*abal ine meluma*) tellingly reflects this precarious situation.

As a result, marital unions have always been fraught with ambivalence. The position of a (newly) married woman in particular is pervaded by ambiguity: for the family of the man, she is a potentially dangerous outsider on whom they depend for the continuation of their lineage; for her own family, she becomes an outsider as well, since she leaves her paternal home and bears children for another family. The Gbigbil adage relating that "a daughter is to be shared" (*mon munka ane komaka*) points to these dual stakes. Never really belonging anywhere, a married woman faces feelings of hostility and solidarity coming from both families (Bonnet 1988; Copet-Rougier 1985; de Thé 1970; Geschiere 1982; Houseman 1988).

In this context, reproduction is explicitly contested. As the number of successors is a main source of social status for both parties, tensions arise around the fact that a married woman, being a descendant of one family, bears descendants for the other. Her relatives can therefore require compensation for the "loss" of their daughter and her childbearing capacities to an unrelated group. This compensation consists of several gifts, social duties, and bride-price payments over time; creating an enduring reciprocal alliance between the lineages, they appease the tensions inherent to exogamous arrangements. While in former times the exchanged commodities were arrows, lances, cowries, food, and cattle, nowadays they include money, red wine, clothes, blankets, food, and small animals. The Gbigbil have clear ideas and ideals about when and how certain presents should be given and reciprocated. Apart from the many small gifts that constantly confirm and conciliate the ambiguous alliance, people mention five major transactions: the wine of presentation, the wine of birth, the money for the mother, *kanako*, and the bride-price.[15]

Ideally, a man (and his relatives) should initiate engagements by introducing himself to a woman's family members with some "wine of presentation" and food, asking for permission to start a "friendship" (*wangang*) with their daughter. After excluding any line of relatedness and assuring their daughter's approval, the woman's relatives then send their daughter for some time to the compound of this man (*keki ibong wangang*), allowing both parties to explore each other's habits.[16] If evaluated positively, the woman can be accepted by her in-laws (*bekil*) as a daughter-in-law (*ngamon*, literally meaning "wife of the child"). Around this acceptance arises a first moment of contestation and conciliation: the woman's brothers will come to ritually demand their sister's return (*atei sa n'abal*) and will agree with the alliance only if the new father-in-law of their sibling sends them home with an acceptable sum of money.

Potential frictions also pervade the relationship between the new ngamon and her in-laws, especially in the first years of marriage. On the one hand, ngamon will be subjected to a wide array of behavioral norms and regulations, prescribing respect, compliance, and diligence. On the other, she can always resort to the intervention of her relatives, publicly express her discontent with her in-laws, or even insult or ridicule them. Tensions manifest themselves particularly in the relationship with the mother-in-law. A newly married woman is obliged to cook in the kitchen of the latter and receives her own kitchen (and, by implication, more independence) only after several years of hard work and strict supervision. The exact moment of this *idang kisin* (literally meaning "traverse of the kitchen") is uncertain and therefore subject to contestation and negotiation; its final happening is celebrated by the woman's relatives, who come to offer new kitchen utensils and food.

The inherent distrust between lineages is clearly revealed around pregnancy and childbirth. Although all the children a married woman bears are supposed to belong to the family of her husband, she will go and deliver with her own relatives. At home, she expects to receive more care and protection than in the family of her husband, where indifference, jealousy, and witchcraft may be omnipresent. After birth, the new mother (*yal*) is allowed to return to her in-laws only once they transfer the "wine of birth" (*medokh meyal*), with which they recompense "the blood that has been spoilt" and acknowledge their descendant(s). On her way back, yal will be accompanied by her own family members, who, upon arrival, will offer another set of gifts to their counterparts.

Hereafter, and irrespective of the number of children borne, a woman's family expects two more transactions before the actual bride-price (*ivoula*). First comes the *monni niaŋa bon* (literally meaning "money for the mother of children"): a sum of money and other gifts given to the woman's mother and maternal aunts to recompense their suffering during the pregnancy, delivery, and education of "their" daughter. Then, people will wait for the kanako, consisting of gifts in duplication: one part goes to the family of the woman's father, the other to the family of her mother.[17] After these two ceremonies, it can take years before the "real" bride-price—a sum of money nowadays set around 100,000 CFA francs, or approximately 150 euros—is collected and paid.[18] The transfer of this bride-price used to be a big public happening, but is nowadays often hidden behind closed doors.

According to norms and expectations, only after the complete payment of the bride-price can a formal marriage certificate—monogamous or polygamous—be signed at the municipality.[19] This certificate offers official acknowledgment of the union and opens the doorway to a religious marriage; only after the conclusion of a (monogamous) civil marriage can a union be confirmed in a church. An *acte de mariage* also protects a woman in case her husband dies. As an "official" widow (*kūs*), she is entitled to stay with her family-in-law, inherit some of her husband's goods, and be buried there when she dies. Without a marriage certificate, a kūs can be sent home or subjected to the principles of the levirate, with the elder brother of the deceased husband inheriting and caring for the latter's wife (or wives).[20] Women without a marriage certificate or without a completed bride-price are generally buried in their natal village. The woman's relatives require the corpse of their daughter as well as a belated bride-price (*doter le corps*) compensating for the "time she has lost" in her marriage and the children she has borne for her husband's lineage. These final contestations and exchanges around women's corpses show that, regardless of the duration of the marriage or the number of children, married women always remain outsiders in the compounds of their husbands.

Although this ideal sequence of marriage transactions is well known to everybody, it does not reflect the actual marital situation in Asung, nor is it likely to be an accurate reflection of what happened in the past. The quantity and quality of bride-price payments seem to have always been subject to change, contestation, and negotiation (Guyer 1986). Studies among the neighboring Beti show how men often preferred to postpone bride-price payments until they had seen a proof of their wives' fertility. At the same time, women appear to have had a considerable behind-the-scenes influence on marriage initiations and negotiations. Furthermore, both men and women would have engaged in sexual relationships before and outside of the prescribed marital framework (de Thé 1970; Houseman 1988; Laburthe-Tolra 1981; Ombolo 1991).

While actual practices have probably always diverged from the norms, they clearly do so today. In contemporary Asung, the expected marriage transactions are often delayed or completely neglected. Men rarely "present" themselves before initiating a relationship with a woman, the "wine of birth" is paid only after many children have been borne, the bigger transactions may just never occur, and marriage certificates may be signed—under the pressure of women and their families—before the bride-price has been paid. Of the 174 surveyed women who considered themselves to be (or have been) married, only 31 percent declared that all marriage transactions had been completed. One-fourth of all married women were in possession of a marriage certificate, and about one-third of these (or 9.5 percent of all married women) had continued the ceremonies in a church.

My informants and several studies in the region (Abega 2007; Johnson-Hanks 2006; Meekers and Calvès 1997; Notermans 1999) attribute the current neglect of marital obligations to the economic crisis that has plagued the country from the late 1980s onward. Financial shortages have severely impacted men's ability to maintain prescribed reciprocities; it would take them longer to assemble the bride-price or to properly provide for their wives and children. Sometimes families are also reluctant to *receive* a bride-price in these economically vulnerable times. They fear to be faced with the impossible task of returning the received goods and money in case the marriage ends. For this reason, they may prefer to let some time pass and ensure themselves of the stability of the relationship before they accept any gifts or money from potential sons-in-law.

In the absence of any marital transactions, many unions in the village are no more than informal "trial marriages" constituted by the living, eating, and sleeping together of two partners. While exchanging food, sex, and money, both partners take time to explore each other's worth: women want to be sure of the good character and financial responsibility of a man and his family before going to "eternalize" there, whereas men wait for a proof of women's fertility before engaging more formally. These "trial marriages" (*ibon*), in which bride-price payments are not yet or hardly initiated, are easily dissolved as soon as one of the partners loses interest; the separation only entails the woman returning to her own family. Local marriages are thus informal, fragile, and flexible forms of cohabitation. This phenomenon is widespread throughout Cameroon; in 2013, a news article in the daily *Cameroon Tribune* noted that, nation-wide, "a disturbing 55 percent of couples are cohabitating [instead of legally married, owing to] the cost of bride price, family and traditional barriers, ignorance and even money to celebrate a legal marriage."[21] Yet, the incidence of informal marriages seems exceptionally high in the East Province (Calvès and Meekers 1999; Notermans 1999).

While "searching for a life," most young people have multiple partners at the same time—sometimes just for sexual or financial rewards, sometimes with the clear aim to try and see whether the relationship could be stabilized into a "marriage" (Calvès and Meekers 1999; Liboko Ndabanga 2001; Njikam Savage 1998). But even in more stable conjugal situations in which partners live together, have several children, and initiated marital transactions, both men and women often maintain extramarital affairs. Men's adulterous behavior is assumed natural and therefore tacitly accepted; women have similar liberties, but their behavior should not become known. These informal relationships might become formalized when a man introduces his lover as a co-wife in his polygynous household (*ival*), or, more rarely, when a woman decides to move in with her "ibon" who seems more promising than her husband. There is no precise dividing line between informal and formal or monogamous and polygamous relationships. As a result, conjugal arrangements are pervaded by secrecy, multiple "bets," skepticism about promises, conflicts (between partners, [potential] co-wives, or affines), and an enormous mobility.

Within this unstable marital terrain, children are borne both within and outside of unions. It is considered acceptable and often even advisable to bear a first child outside of marriage. The presence of a child proves one's fertility and is expected to increase marriage chances in uncertain times when men do not easily engage.[22] Whether their first birth leads to marriage or not, many Gbigbil women (and their families) express a clear wish to bear their second and following children *dans un foyer* (in a household). To bear "every child with another man" is not deemed honorable (*digne*). It exposes a woman's multiple sexual activities and might make men unwilling to take responsibility in the event that they are appointed as the father of a pregnancy. Furthermore, if a man *is* willing to engage, the fact that there are already children from different relationships might complicate the marriage arrangement. Men seldom accept to bear the burden of caring for someone else's "blood." Especially sons are rarely allowed to grow up (and, by implication, stay) in the compound of another lineage. Daughters are easier to accept; they will finally leave the compound for marriage and might even offer brideprice rewards in the long run.

As pregnancies are conceived both within and outside of marriage, the right to children is contested. The official Gbigbil kinship idiom is patrilineal: although procreative roles of both father and mother are acknowledged, children—containing blood of both parents—are said to ultimately belong to the lineage of their father, provided that he paid the bride-price for his wife.[23] However, since men are often neglectful or unable to transfer the demanded payments, in practice their paternity is not self-evident. Opinions about their right to children in the absence of a bride-price differ: some people cling to the bride-price payments as a precondition of paternity, while most others just demand a man's acknowledgment of his paternity and his (financial) care of mother and child(ren) during and after pregnancy. This care encompasses the provision of a layette (*bidəl abial*, literally meaning "clothes of birth"), a package of baby clothes, diapers, towels, baby oils, and powders that costs 7,500 CFA francs (around 11 euros). This layette seems to have almost replaced the bride-price in establishing a rightful claim on one's descendants. When men do *not* recognize their paternity or assume financial responsibilities, however, women bear and raise their children in their own families. Negligent partners who come to claim their children after six years—when children are supposed to move to their father's family—are often heavily fined or even deprived of their children, who are now perceived to belong to the woman's patrilineage.

Next to claiming the children of their daughter *after* birth, maternal families may ask for more descendants *before* a woman gets involved in a conjugal relationship. Besides being a much wanted proof of fertility, first pregnancies often serve the needs for offspring of the woman's own family. The current flexibility of sexual and marital arrangements offers room for maneuvering to women (and their families), who can explicitly deny paternity or refuse the help of the genitor in order to undermine his claims on the child. Further, many women send their children to be raised by their own family members (preferably a mother or sister) in order to mediate the claims of paternity by their partner and the demands for children by their relatives. More than one-third of 287 surveyed women stated that, contrary to prescribed norms, their child(ren) resided within their maternal rather than paternal families. These exceptions to the patrilineal rule show that kinship relations, like marital configurations, are fraught by discrepancies between ideals and reality.

Aside from all these local social dynamics, national and international forces also shape the landscape through which Gbigbil people navigate on a daily basis. The rest of this chapter will explore the domain of (reproductive) health policies and interventions. As we will see, this "terrain" is also pervaded by multiple discrepancies between ideals and realities.

The Promises and Problems of Public Health

Cameroon used to be one of the African countries whose potential for economic development was highly praised after independence. Its abundance of natural resources and a fairly strong position on the international market, as well as the health infrastructures left by German, British, and French colonizers, inspired hopes for a future in which the country would self-sufficiently provide for the economic and sanitary well-being of its inhabitants. With almost none of this optimism left today, people yearn for the promising postcolonial days they lived under President Ahidjo, offering them fairly well organized developments and state-sponsored services. The nostalgia of hindsight and the increasing indeterminacy of foresight make them present the free hospital services of those times as qualitatively better and less pervaded by corruption than current care. However, this idealization of the past tends to ignore the poor management and corruption that Cameroon's health system has long known (Médard 2001).

While early colonial health services were particularly focused on the army and the European population—and thus largely conglomerated in urban centers—after the Second World War new ideas about health and development inspired the expansion of services to rural areas in Cameroon. Health came to be viewed as an essential element and precondition of development; a healthy population would be indispensable for a healthy labor force and thus the development (*mise en valeur*) of the country. The resulting increase of expenditures on health (from 12.2 percent in 1940 to 24.6 percent in 1945) allowed for the development and improvement of fixed infrastructures, as well as the creation of itinerant health services. Mobile teams entered rural areas, such as the one in which the Gbigbil resided, for systematic medical screenings and massive vaccination interventions from the 1950s onward (Leh 1987; Ngono 2005).[24]

After independence in 1960, health was one of the sectors that figured prominently in the five-year plans that guided the process of nation building. However, these development policies lacked intra- and intersectorial coherence and rendered the Cameroonian health system vertically organized. Largely in the hands of former colonizers and international organizations, the approach was mainly curative and informed by absolute priorities—for example, the fight against high child mortality or endemic diseases such as sleeping sickness, tuberculosis, and leprosy. Consequently, health services remained disproportionately distributed over the country and inaccessible to those in neglected areas (Eto 2005; Leh 1987; Maynard 2004).[25]

This unequal approach was gradually altered after the Alma Ata conference in 1978, during which the need for "health for all by the year 2000" was expressed. Recognizing health as a human right and a precondition for economic and social development, the conference members stated that primary health care should be accessible—economically, geographically, and culturally—to everybody. Health care should further be explicitly *community based* and *preventive* as well as curative. Cameroon adopted this primary health care approach in 1982. Its major aim was to provide continuous rather than intermittent health services, which would be integrated at the village level. However, despite the successes with regard to certain health indicators in the initial years after implementation of the new approach, the economic crisis in Cameroon since the mid-1980s severely disrupted and curtailed many government programs, including those in public health. The national health budget dropped from 800 billion CFA francs in 1987–1988 to 572 billion CFA francs in 1991–1992; its share of the GDP decreased from 5.2 percent in 1989 to 4.4 percent in 1991 (Owono Essomba et al. 1993). Numerous problems have since been noted with regard to the execution of the primary health care approach—pertaining not only to the health services, but also to the community level and its relationship with the existing health structures.

In order to correct these insufficiencies, the primary health care approach was redefined first in 1985 after the World Health Organization (WHO)-sponsored conference of Lusaka and again in 1987 after the Harare conference and the Bamako Initiative, where two major strategies to "rationalize" primary health care were launched: cofinancing and comanagement. First, a system of "cost recovery" was introduced in which patients would be required to pay for the health services in order to increase the system's efficiency.[26] Second, a decentralization of decision-making power into local hands was proposed, supposedly leading to higher quality of care and greater participation of communities in the (financial) management of sanitary services. The partnership between local communities and the health care structure would be further reinforced by the instauration of community agents and committees mediating between the two parties.

The resulting "reorientation of primary health care"—formally adopted in 1993—entailed a complete reorganization of Cameroon's sanitary map. The health care system was formally organized into a pyramidal structure consisting of three major levels: central (national), intermediate (provincial), and peripheral (local health districts, subdivided into geographically demarcated "health areas" such as the one surrounding Asung).[27] The latter, representing the interface between the local population and governmental services, was supposed to carry out essential health services in a self-sufficient and integrated way, with considerable participation of the inhabitants of the health districts. Offering a "minimal package of care"—consisting of curative, preventive, and promotional activities—the Integrated Health Centers (Centres de Santé Intégré), as they were called, would now have to refer only difficult cases to the provincial or central level (Ministère de la Santé Publique Cameroun 1993a).

These elaborate revisions of the health care structure did not lead to the envisaged results. As the economic crisis continued to ravage the country, several international attempts to develop the national economy and reduce macroeconomic inequalities inhibited the process of health reformation. First, in 1989, Structural Adjustment Programs were introduced, which drastically cut public expenditure on health. Not only did health workers suddenly see their salaries reduced by half, but they also faced an increased workload as the influx of newly trained health personnel was put on a hold. Both the health care system and the health status of Cameroonians deteriorated dramatically as a result (Kamdoum 1994). Later, in 2000, the admission of Cameroon to the Highly Indebted Poor Countries Initiative made its health policies even more dependent on international conditions and standards. "Health" came to be defined as one of the sectors (next to education, agriculture, and infrastructure) that would have to be made more operational with regard to human, material, and financial resources. Yet, the 2001–2015 Health Sector Strategy and the National Plan of Sanitary Development for 2011–2015, which guided this process, were subject to endless updates as problems with meeting the objectives were continuously anticipated.[28]

With governmental influence gradually fading away, many nongovernmental organizations, private enterprises, and confessional establishments have come to play a prominent role in the domain of primary health care in Cameroon. The private nonprofit sector currently provides 40 percent of the overall national health care; it is largely dominated by faith-based providers (Boulenger, Barten, and Criel 2014). Owing to its long history in the country, the (Catholic and Protestant) confessional sector has even created its own sanitary map. The Catholics have divided the country into autonomous dioceses with an important network of operational sanitary establishments, of which thirty-three can be found in the East Province and one in Asung's neighboring village of Kamandjom.[29] They train health personnel, order drugs, and negotiate with the Ministry of Health. Although drugs at these missionary and other private clinics—even the allegedly "noncommercial" ones—are often relatively expensive, the mere *presence* of medicines as well as the better services leads many people, like the Gbigbil, to resort to these health centers (Kamdoum 1994; Médard 2001; van der Geest 1982b).

This amalgam of public, private, national, and international interventions has contributed to an enormous "balkanization" of the current health situation in the country. Without much coordination, all parties launch different strategies, priorities, and zones of intervention. To this come the many informal activities within local medical terrains. Because of the drastic deterioration of both their own financial situations and public health services, people increasingly resort to "indigenous" practitioners (of whom 804 are registered in the East Province) or to self-medication. Others venture themselves on the informal drug market, where they find counterfeit products—mostly coming from Nigeria and sold in small shops or by street vendors—as well as biomedical medicines from formal institutions, illicitly appropriated and privately sold by health personnel (Eto 2005; Gruenais 2001; Kamdoum 1994; Kamtcha 2004; van der Geest 1982a).

Like Cameroon's economic sector, the health sector witnesses a complex interrelation between informal and formal domains (Geschiere and Konings 1993; Niger-Thomas 2000). "Indigenous" healers increasingly use innovative and biomedical symbols in order to advertise a "veritable African tradition"; Chinese therapies create new hopes and confidence; biomedical staff construct informal neighborhood offices in order to ensure "proximity care"; and the unemployed find in the drug business a new way of making their own living, while sick people rely on it for their self-medication. Ironically, this informal health sector seems to attain the goal that remains unachieved by formal public health strategies: namely, to reach and satisfy the needs of the local population.

To conclude, the health situation in Cameroon is extremely dynamic and characterized by internal contradictions. While there has been an increasing focus on de jure decentralization and financial autonomy, de facto all levels of the health pyramid system are pervaded by centralization, bureaucratization, patrimonialism, and corruption. Rather than the anticipated de jure community participation in the 178 health districts and 3,214 public health facilities that currently cover the country, de facto people increasingly turn to illicit and cheaper alternatives within this diverse health terrain. This "profound crisis of the Cameroonian health system," as Médard (2001) has called it, has certainly been exacerbated by the economic adversities since the mid-1980s, but not exclusively so; it also seems a historically situated, structural problem. It has therefore also affected the terrain of reproductive health care in Cameroon.

Reevaluating Reproductive Health

Within the pyramidal structure outlined above, all three health care levels are supposed to offer reproductive health services. Peripheral health centers should offer maternal and child care as an integrative part of the "minimum package of care," specific mother and child care centers in all provinces provide family planning services and aim to reduce maternal and infant mortality, and major cities host clinics for sexually transmitted diseases and high-risk pregnancies (Ako et al. 2003). This omnipresence of reproductive health services is, however, largely informed by recently formulated international targets; in the past, priorities regarding the reproduction of the Cameroonian population used to be different.

As mentioned before, colonists already expressed concerns regarding the low density and uneven distribution of the colony's population. Especially the East Province, in which the Gbigbil were situated, had a very low population count, exacerbated by the high infertility levels in this region. In order to bring economic development (*mise en valeur*) to this province and the rest of the colony, measures were taken to fight the underpopulation (*sous-peuplement*)—seen as the main reason for the underdevelopment (*sous-développement*)—and multiply the number of African producers. These measures consisted not only of medical and educational interventions trying to eradicate the spread of epidemics, but also of the distribution of explicitly pronatalist slogans such as "operation 10 million inhabitants by 1960" (Feldman-Savelsberg 2002; Geschiere 1982; Gubry and Wautelet 1993; Ngo Bell 1990).

After independence in 1960, this line of thinking continued. Whereas the first five-year development plan reiterated the colonial concerns about the unequal distribution and underutilization of the workforce, the third plan ten years later (1971–1975) explicitly mentioned the desirability of demographic growth for productivity and the exploitation of the territory.[30] This growth was encouraged through unequivocal government measures: civil servants with a large family profited from family allowances and tax reductions;[31] parents of twelve children or more were offered special medals for their "contribution to the nation"; the media and official discourses praised the high proportion of youngsters in the population as the "spearhead" and "vital force" of the nation; midwives were massively trained in order to reduce infant and maternal mortality; and any limitation of fertility was legally restricted by a 1969 law prohibiting the publicity and sale of contraceptives, as well as by penal laws repressing abortion and infanticide.[32] Cameroon's population expanded. Owing to a decline in mortality rates—with those for infants dropping from 190 in 1,000 in 1950 to 88 in 1,000 in 1987—and a rise of the average fertility rate to more than six children per woman, the number of inhabitants almost doubled in thirty years, from 4.5 million in 1950 to 8.5 million in the early 1980s (Ako et al.

2003; Bahanag 2003; Feldman-Savelsberg 2002; Ngo Bell 1990; Tantchou and Wilson 2000).

Meanwhile, the international community started to worry about the enormous population growth in developing countries like Cameroon, which would negatively affect the natural environment and socioeconomic development. From the 1974 World Population Conference in Bucharest onward, explicit recommendations were made to reduce population growth rates in these countries. Not surprisingly, Cameroon initially rejected these ideas and propositions. In reaction to the international plea for birth control, the government stated that it would consider family planning only as "a synonym of birth spacing with the aim to preserve mother and child health" (Ako et al. 2003; Nseke 2002; Sala-Diakanda 2000). The first inclusion and promotion of "responsible parenthood" in the fifth five-year plan (1981–1986) was still precarious and sometimes explicitly contested (Bahanag 2003). Only from the sixth five-year plan onward were demographic variables incorporated into the country's development strategies. Presenting this plan at the National Assembly, President Paul Biya declared:

> I would like at this point to draw the attention of Cameroonians of both sexes to the economic and social consequences of an unplanned increase in the birth rate. Procreation, albeit a basic human right, can and must be controlled. The purpose here is not to discard our beliefs, practices and customs in this regard, but rather to increasingly strive for the systematic promotion and institutionalization of planned and responsible parenthood. (Commission Nationale de la Population Cameroun 1993: 27)

This change in attitude was accompanied by a gradual relaxation of the law prohibiting the sale and publicity of contraceptives,[33] as well as the creation of a National Population Commission in 1985 that would assist the Cameroonian government in the definition and orientation of a population policy.[34]

The ensuing National Population Policy was adopted in 1992. It stipulated people's rights to "freely decide on the number of children they may wish to have" as well as their responsibility to ensure the future welfare of these children.[35] In the same year, with the support of the United Nations Population Fund (UNFPA), family planning was integrated in existing maternal and child health services. The latter, in turn, became an essential element of public health after the "reorientation of primary health care" one year later. All levels of the pyramidal system were from now on supposed to "ameliorate and promote the well-being of mother and child in order to reduce the morbidity and mortality rates that remain high in this group" (Commission Nationale de la Population Cameroun 1993: 41). Therefore, contraceptives were included on the national list of essential drugs, policy guidelines were standardized, and training sessions were organized for family planning service deliverers in 1996.

Despite these formal revisions, the Cameroonian government remained rather reluctant to fully adopt international definitions of and guidelines for reproductive health. Only after its admission to the Highly Indebted Poor Countries Initiative in the year 2000, which increased international surveillance and pressure, did it develop various comprehensive reproductive health plans and policies, inspired by the Millennium Development Goals.[36] An updated version of the National Population Policy (2001) and the Reproductive Health component of the 2001–2015 Health Sector Strategy now stress "the promotion of quality reproductive health services, notably for the mastery of procreation" and the fight against sexually transmissible infections and HIV/AIDS. Rather than focusing only on mothers and children, these documents also pay particular attention to the reproductive health status of men, adolescents, and old people.

With policies becoming more and more inclusive, abortions have increasingly been mentioned as a major reproductive health problem in the country. While the first National Population Policy of 1992 stated that "teenage pregnancies, abandoned children and illegal and life-threatening abortions have become ever increasing and severe social problems," nothing tangible was done to tackle the problem—no legal adjustments, no sanitary provisions. In its revised version of 2001, the policy explicitly underscores the need to "reduce the number of unwanted and early pregnancies as well as provoked abortions caused by adolescents," and to recognize postabortion care (PAC) as an essential element of reproductive health care (Ministère de la Santé Publique Cameroun 2001a, 2001b).[37] Yet, no concrete strategies are proposed to attain these goals.

An actual implementation of the policy seems hampered by article 337 in the penal law of Cameroon, which almost invariably punishes abortion with imprisonment or heavy fines.[38] The two exceptional circumstances under which abortions can be lawfully performed concern situations in which the pregnancy resulted from convicted rape, or is perceived by at least three professionals to endanger the life of the mother. As most pregnancies do not fit these categories, in practice women can resort only to clandestine and often unsafe means to abort them: they use dangerous methods themselves, seek help from indigenous healers, or illegally undergo dilation and curettage (D&C) procedures after bribing biomedical staff at a considerable cost. The numerous unsafe abortions would contribute to an estimated 20 to 40 percent of the growing maternal mortality rate in the country.

A more integrative approach to the abortion problem remains complicated, partly because of the constitutive role played by the confessional sector in Cameroon's health care system. Despite their long and active history of providing maternal and child health services, Catholic congregations remain reticent when it comes to family planning and abortion. Most of them promote only natural means of fertility control through abstinence or calculation of the menstrual cycle. Protestant churches have been more liberal in their visions; many Presbyterian hospitals in Cameroon do provide reproductive health and family planning services. Islamic leaders, to the contrary, are noted to occasionally oppose educational programs for youngsters or women's use of contraception (Ngo Bell 1990; Sala-Diakanda 2000; Tantchou and Wilson 2000).

This multiplicity of political, moral, and juridical discourses surrounding reproductive health in Cameroon has resulted in a complex situation in which rhetoric is at odds with the practical circumstances in the country. While the general approach toward population matters turned from explicitly pronatalist to "supportive to family planning," in practice access to birth control methods remains hampered by legislative and practical barriers (such as laws prescribing the sale of contraceptives by pharmacies only, de facto requests for the authorization of the partner, and stringent criteria for more permanent contraceptive measures such as sterilization).[39] While maternal and child health services became an integrative part of primary health care, their practical accessibility and quality remain fairly low.[40] While the concept of reproductive health was finally included in the revised National Population Policy and numerous health strategies in the country, the latest Demographic and Health Survey of 2011 shows little reduction in infant, child, and maternal mortality rates as well as an alarming propagation of the HIV/AIDS pandemic.[41] While postabortion care is now mentioned as an element of reproductive health services, the underlying dynamics that motivate women to resort to (unsafe) abortion methods in the first place remain ignored. And while different stakeholders share the attention to "hyperfertility," they tend to forget the high—although drastically reduced—number of women having to deal with infertility and pregnancy interruptions.[42] Clearly, there is a huge gap between Cameroon's policy priorities—reflecting economic dependencies and international power relations—and the actual reproductive health situations and stakes in the local terrains. The latter will be further explored in the rest of this book.

Pregnancies
in Practice

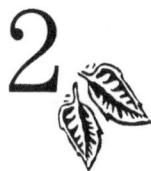

2

DIANNE IS SITTING IN HER KITCHEN, waiting for the cassava to cook in the pot on the fire. While I am playing with her seven-month-old daughter, Joëlle, on my lap, Dianne starts moving uneasily on the bamboo bed opposite me. Hesitantly she tells me there is something she would like to ask. "I have been waiting for my period for a few days now. Normally I start bleeding every thirteenth of the month, but this month I didn't see anything. How is this possible? Do you think I am pregnant?" Somewhat bedazzled I inquire about her menstrual cycle during her current breastfeeding period, and she tells me that the principle of "not menstruating while nursing" does not apply to her. Smiling shyly and bending her head, she adds that the local norm of abstaining from sexual intercourse during this period also does not work for her and her husband Baudouin. Although they try to avoid intercourse during her fertile days, Dianne reflects, "It could be this kind of accident that happens when you don't enter a car because you are afraid of accidents, but then you slip and sprain your ankle while walking. You see how accidents happen? You try to avoid them, but there is always a risk." Together we conclude that she also risks being pregnant now.

I ask Dianne if she has already discussed the matter with Baudouin. She tells me that she did and that her husband is very proud to know that she missed her period. Since they have only one daughter together, he is eagerly waiting for another baby—preferably a son. She herself, however, thinks it is far too early for another pregnancy. It could endanger the life of her nursing daughter. "A pregnancy will spoil my milk, and Joëlle might even die![1] She should first reach fifteen months before a new pregnancy enters. A gap of two years between two children is good. Both will survive." Next to worries about Joëlle's well-being, Dianne expresses concerns about her own status in the village. The thought of being seen with a big belly in front and with Joëlle attached to her back—something that would surely give rise to animated gossip and public scorn—is almost unbearable. "I don't sleep anymore, or I dream that I see my period. Sometimes I just wear sanitary towels in my underwear, hoping that some bloodstains will appear on it, but I don't see anything. If this turns out to be a pregnancy, I will search for remedies that will evacuate the blood that is now obstructed by the pregnancy." Since she once almost lost her life while trying to remove an advanced pregnancy with a needle, Dianne has decided to act as quickly as possible this time.

A few days later we meet again and discuss the matter at hand. Visibly troubled, Dianne informs me that there is still no sign of a period. When I ask her what the next step will be, she says that she intends to visit the hospital's pharmacist. During a coincidental encounter earlier that week, she had asked him to help her out. Although he had initially refused, he had eventually suggested that she buy some Nivaquine pills;[2] since he has a stock at home, she could just come and take some pills there, secretly. Dianne sighs. "Oh Erica, just pray for me that the thing that we talked about doesn't stay and that it will leave quickly with those pills. I will let you know as soon as I see the blood." And so it happens. When I meet Dianne a few days later at the market, she grabs my hand and whispers, "It has come." Visibly relieved, she assures me that all she will do now is take good care of her little Joëlle.

Vividly remembering this happy ending of a worrisome period, I am rather surprised when Dianne tells me one month later that she really regrets having taken those pills. Probed to elaborate further, she says, "In the end, it was not even a pregnancy. One can never know, but I am quite sure it was only a troubled period. After all, my husband and I had constantly avoided a pregnancy. We accurately counted my cycle and it was almost impossible I would conceive. It is only this time that I think it might be a real pregnancy. Although I talked a lot to my husband, he did not want to listen to me." Even more confused I ask her if she means that she again missed her period this month. She relates how Baudouin had forced her to have intercourse during her fertile days and that she will have to wait and see if she will menstruate later this month. She does not. Without telling her husband, she buys some Nivaquine pills, which again prove effective. In the months that follow, Dianne continues to share her insecurities with me every time her period is due. When I leave the field, Joëlle's first birthday has just passed. I ask Dianne what would happen if she were to get pregnant after my departure. Smilingly shrugging her shoulders she says, "It is God who sends children. I would not refuse it. Joëlle is old enough now to allow my belly to grow."

Just like many other Gbigbil women that I came to know when I lived in Asung, Dianne involved me in the uncertain period around missed menses and potential pregnancies. Like the others, she constantly redefined her notions of menstruation, missed period, "troubled" period, and conception—as well as the desirability of each of these events at specific moments. The very conceptualization of a pregnancy seemed flexible and negotiable. This chapter will highlight the reasons for this flexibility and explore its repercussions on women's management of their pregnancies. A review of local constructs of menstruation, conception, embryology, and delivery will show that not only moments such as the ones faced by Dianne, but also many other reproductive processes in Gbigbil women's lives are uncertain, flexible, and contingent. How do women deal with such reproductive indeterminacies in their everyday lives? And how do they navigate Asung's social and medical terrains during the uncertain antenatal period? Answering these questions, this chapter maps the landscape of fertility in which Gbigbil women's navigation of "wasted wombs" should be situated. Only when we know how reproduction is generally imagined and enacted can we start exploring what it means to lose or interrupt a pregnancy. So let us begin with the very beginning: the gift of fertility.

Female Physiology and Fertility

Though Dianne repeatedly wished to evacuate what she thought would eventually become a pregnancy, she also assured me that she did not refuse the children God would send to her. When talking about her aspirations for the future, she expressed the desire to eternalize in Baudouin's household and bear as many children as possible—even ten, if God wanted her to. In the end, Gbigbil women like Dianne would say, it is God (Zambe) who decides to send a child to a woman or not, whatever her own childbearing intentions at that moment. "L'homme propose, Dieu dispose" (Man proposes, God disposes) is an expression that they often invoked in this respect.

The general capacity to reproduce is also seen as a divine gift. God gives women their reproductive organs and blesses them (or not) with "the blood for childbearing." Every woman is thought to have a predestined number of children (*mizəng mibon*) on her "cords of children" (*mikol mibon*) in the womb (*kombe*), waiting for God to decide when and to what extent they will develop.[3] The cords of children were often compared to chains. Indeed, the word *zang* denominating the children (*bon*) who await their maturation on the cords is also used for the beads of a necklace. Others equate the Gbigbil word for cords (*mikol*) with the French word for fallopian tubes (*trompes*), while leaving its function as residence for children-to-be unaltered. Although all women are believed to be endowed with such cords—or fallopian tubes, for that matter—not everybody is lucky to have "the blood for childbearing." Some might end up permanently infertile, while others are only intermittently sent children by God—an affliction called *abial kok*, or "the childbirth of a giraffe." By locating their reproductive capacities within the natural (blood) or supernatural (God) realm, Gbigbil women portray fertility as an unalterable affair; what resonates through their depictions is the inherent uncertainty and unpredictability of reproduction—not only its endowment, but also its onset, its development, and its outcomes.

Although God's plans can never be known by human beings, there are several ways in which women's destinies can be (temporarily) revealed. In cases of infertility, or abial kok, women can consult diviners to find out whether they (still) "have children in the belly" or not. Such healers may even reveal the conditions under which these children can come into development. Likewise, I heard several accounts of dreams in which dead relatives predict fertility outcomes and announce ways to achieve them. This happened to mama Stéphanie, whose dead father had proclaimed in a dream that she would first bear two girls out of wedlock and give them to her own family—which, ultimately, she did. It also happened to mama Rosie's paternal aunt, who was told by her dead father to rub saliva on the belly of her brother's wife (mama Rosie's mother), which would result in a pregnancy of a girl to whom she was to give her own name: Rosie. The realizations of such dreams show again how the fertility of Gbigbil women is perceived to be predestined and subjected to both divine and ancestral approval.[4]

This does not mean, however, that such ideas of spiritual endowment render women fatalistic or turn them into passive carriers of their pregnancies. To the contrary: almost paradoxically, women may invoke exactly this idea of predestination to justify their fertility regulation and management practices. Especially when they have already borne at least one child, this proof of "having children in the belly" gives them considerable room for maneuver. My neighbor Dorine, for instance, was a nineteen-year-old mother of one four-year-old daughter, who longed to postpone childbearing. One day, she uncovered her breast to me to show the stretch marks that had appeared there during her pregnancy. Calling them "lines of children," she argued that they would be visible only on the skin of women "with many children in their bellies." Dorine's visual proof and expressed conviction of her endowment of fertility seemed to appease the clash between the social pressure to bear another child and her own refusal to do so. Since she could show that God had given her "the blood of childbearing," she claimed to feel "no need to rush" and to have leeway to prevent conception for the time being. Thus, the idea of predestination does not inhibit women from exerting certain kinds of agency in their daily reproductive lives; it often *supports* them in doing so.

One concrete manifestation of divine endowment that is central to women's reproductive management is menstruation. Asked about the reason behind their monthly periods, all Gbigbil women invariably answered that it was God who had decided that women should menstruate in order to bear children. With the onset of menses, a girl's body turns from a dry state into a wet, mature condition. Women's mature bodies are regulated by a normal flow of blood, which can become blocked by conception; in fact, every menstruation is considered a missed chance for a pregnancy. If no conception has occurred, the body will open itself at the moment of menstruation and evacuate the blood, as well as the sperm of last month's intercourses that have not resulted in a pregnancy. Apart from a marker of womanhood and possible motherhood, menstruation is therefore considered a regulatory mechanism of the body, which "removes all the dirt" and keeps the female body healthy.

Though women believe that this regulatory flow is a natural process created by God, they might give it a helping hand. From time to time, they "wash the stomach" (*isŏ abum*) by drinking or vaginally administering herbal remedies, or by resorting to biomedical injections or dilation and curettage (D&C) services.[5] In this way, they aim to remove the extra "dirt" (*bĭt*) that accumulates over time, to prevent the blockage of fallopian tubes, to regain regular menses, or to encourage conception in a clean and healthy body. Other interventions aim to regulate the workings of the "women's worm" (*song bunka*), believed to wander around in the belly and cause menstrual (and premenstrual) pains with its teeth. In normal conditions, this worm is supposed to open its mouth once a month around the same date, after which blood is released and menstruation induced. Daniëlle explained:

There are different sorts of worms. There is the bad worm that causes miscarriage, but there is also the "worm of childbirth." That's uniquely for your menstruation. When you are about to see your period, it will bite you in the lower abdomen. As soon as you have your menstruation, it stops and does not hurt anymore. If you would get pregnant then, you wouldn't even have problems. It doesn't evacuate your pregnancy. It's not too bad to have this kind of worm. It's even normal.

The workings of the women's worm become *abnormal*, however, when blood is abundant, thick, darkly colored, or accompanied by a lot of pain (*isōki*). Here, the bad form of the women's worm is suspected to be at work; the condition becomes pathologized. The extreme pain it causes in the lower abdomen is said to make women scream out loud before and during menstruation—something that is highly unusual in a setting where women are not supposed to publicly express their pain. Human intervention in these so-called troubled or painful periods is deemed indispensable and can take place only "indigenously" (à l'*indigène*) with local herbs, as treatment at the hospital is thought to aggravate the situation. This condition affects many women during their reproductive trajectories; almost half (48 percent) of all 290 women who participated in my survey indicated to have suffered from this worm at least once in their lives (see Appendix VI).

Thus, despite the perception that menstruation is a natural process created by God, Gbigbil women constantly observe, evaluate, and regulate the frequency, color, smell, thickness, volume, or pain level of their periods. Most menstrual regulation practices serve yet another goal: the evacuation of "what could become a pregnancy." "Washing the stomach" then becomes a means to prevent the "crossing" of sperm and blood, and thus the eventual formation of a pregnancy. Such postconceptional inducements are supported by local embryological notions that portray gestational development as a very gradual process—rendering the initial stages of a pregnancy ambiguous and explicitly manageable.

Filling with Force: Gbigbil Embryology

At the end of menstruation, a small amount of blood is believed to stay behind in the woman's vagina and "wait for the pregnancy." It is at this point that conception is perceived most likely to occur; since the female body is still in an open state, it is very receptive to men's semen (*medom*). However, this does not always automatically mean that a pregnancy (*abum*; also the word for belly) results if semen enters at this moment. Although bodily conditions are most favorable to conception now, its actual happening remains uncertain and ultimately dependent on God's will. As one woman once made clear, "If God wants you to be infertile, you can make love as much as you want, but you won't conceive. The sperm enters, but it will be evacuated by your menstrual blood and by vaginal secretions."

However, if both physical and metaphysical conditions are favorable to conception, the opening in the woman's body will close as soon as the semen has passed it. The flow of menstrual blood is now blocked and will mix with the semen in order to gradually "form a pregnancy" (*ayadīm abum*). Since sperm is considered a derivative of a man's blood, Gbigbil people often talk about the mixing of "bloods" at this point. Here a third condition (next to metaphysical accordance and physical susceptibility) comes into play to ensure a successful conception: the compatibility of the man's and the woman's blood. These are conceptualized as groups A, B, and C or as having different "strengths." The blood of men, youngsters, and Africans is stronger than the blood of women, the elderly, or white people. Problems in conception are believed to occur when blood strengths are too disparate or blood groups dissimilar.[6]

Only the mixture of two compatible bloods will form a small ball of blood in the vagina. Some compare this ball to an egg (*atiə mon*); others maintain that it is no more than a mix of fluids (*aginene medii*: "it is still water"; *medii medii*: "water water").[7] Indeed, to say in Gbigbil that a woman's pregnancy is in the beginning phase of gestation is to say that "she has water in her body" (*anene medii a nyol*). Tellingly, to "wash the stomach" at this stage is translated as simply "evacuating the water" (*mevā medii*). Rather than considered an *interruption* of a pregnancy, it is explained as the *prevention* of further development into a pregnancy. Women like Dianne can "evacuate water" on a monthly basis, if that is deemed necessary, without feeling any moral scruples. What they remove is not an established pregnancy yet; at most, what is in the process of being "formed" could possibly end up being a pregnancy.

Not surprisingly, when asked to draw the development of a pregnancy on an empty body map, Gbigbil women were often at a loss about what to draw at one month gestation. Many of them were inclined to give the body map immediately back to me, asking rhetorically how they could draw "something that is not yet anything." Probed to designate what they meant by "not yet anything" they would then try to depict a mass of liquids. Some women, more or less influenced by Christian notions of immediate life after conception, acknowledged the potentiality of this liquid ball to become a person. They assured me that the movements of the developing ball could already be felt in the lower abdomen during this first month of pregnancy. Whether perceived as a complete "void" or as a potential human being, this "loose" substance that could potentially become a child (*mon*, pl. *bon*) is called *zəng mon* as long as it does not display clear human forms. Zəng mon slowly ascends from the vagina into the uterus and intensifies its movements around two or three months of gestation. Gradually, the ball is transformed into a lizard-like creature with a tail in a sitting position. All limbs are thought to be present, but "the child is not yet well formed" (*atəka kombā*).

When exactly the child *will* be formed is unknown; the process of forming a human-like mon depends mainly on the force of the blood of both the father and the mother—a force that is in itself variable over a lifetime. A zəng mon of parents with strong blood develops quickly; those inheriting weak blood transform themselves more slowly into mon. Of constitutive value is the blood that surrounds, nourishes, fills, and protects zəng mon until it is completely formed. Further, informants who believed that zəng mon resides in the amniotic sac (*akonnā*)—often simply called "bag of water" or "plastic bag" in French—attributed the same nourishing functions to the amniotic water. Next to these liquids, zəng mon is also thought to be fed via the umbilical cord, which transfers the mother's ingested food directly, via the bowels or via her blood. Finally, zəng mon is thought to feed itself through an opening in the head, which during birth transforms into the delicate fontanel. The food that a mother ingests passes directly through this opening into the fetus's body and forms the first black stools (*ikokogli*) of the newborn baby.

In this developing phase, women are encouraged to have regular sexual intercourse with the father of the growing fetus. Not only will this "keep the route open," but, more importantly, his sperm (i.e., his transformed blood) is deemed constitutive of zəng mon's developing body. The child will strongly resemble his father if it has been regularly "fed" by his sperm—especially if this "blood" is very strong. In this respect, I heard several women say that "it is the man who gives the child" or "it is the man who has to work most for the pregnancy." Sexual intercourse with men other than the genitor—or the "mixing of the pregnancy" (*apulă abum*)—should at all times be avoided; the child would hate the smell of their semen and refuse to descend during childbirth.

This essential contribution of the father to the successful completion of the pregnancy has been noted by other studies as well (Aboubakar 2008; Beninguissé 2003; Erny 1988; Godelier 1992; Krumeich 1994; Scheper-Hughes and Lock 1987; Tsala Tsala 1996). It is often interpreted as the ultimate expression of patriarchal discourses claiming men's superiority and women's dependence on men. Yet, the perceived necessity of intercourse for paternal resemblance should also be situated within a local context of sexual flexibility and marital instability, rendering paternity uncertain and contested. In such a context, the appearance of a baby has become an important indicator of who must be the father—and by implication, who must be responsible for, and can claim rights over, the child (see further Chapter 4). Women who went to school or learned from their own experiences may, however, dismiss this indispensability of the genitor's semen—or of substitutes such as the gluey *mbol* sauce, ingested by pregnant women when their partner is absent. Through such a dismissal, they often try to justify their own "multipartenariat," which would otherwise be labeled as adulterous or strictly forbidden by mamas in the village.

Even when all human features are formed and zəng mon has transformed itself into mon—whenever that may be—the process of growing and filling continues. This process is now essential to provide mon with force (*ngul*). In this second phase of fetal development, which informants broadly estimate to start somewhere between three and five months after conception, the child moves toward the upper belly, facing the spine, where the placenta is believed to be stuck. Here, mon becomes almost a separate agent leading its own life: it walks around, sleeps, plays, urinates, refuses food or asks for it—all of which can be directly felt by the mother. The mother's food intake is now, next to her continuous supply of blood, deemed increasingly crucial to fill mon with force, while sexual intercourse is considered less necessary as the child is already fully developed. Intercourse is even forbidden toward the end of pregnancy since the "excess of sperm" may stick to the newborn baby and shamefully expose one's sexual activities upon birth.

Only when mon is filled with a certain level of force will he or she be able to live outside of the uterus. Some attain this level after five or six months, others only at seven or eight months, and the very slow ones or twins may even need ten or eleven months. Once viability and life force abound, it is mon who decides when a pregnancy comes to term (*tun abum*), by initiating childbirth with his or her own force—rupturing the placenta with the nails and subsequently scratching its way out. Thus, the final point of a "normal" pregnancy does not depend on a fixed time frame but varies according to the parents' blood strength and thereby a child's development pace. Asked to draw a seven-month pregnancy on a body map, all informants decided to draw mon's head turned downward "since some children can be born already by this time." One of these drawings reveals the hesitation and uncertainty surrounding gestational timing; after having drawn the head upward, my informant corrected the fetal position when bystanders reminded her of the possibility of a quickly developed mon with strong blood.

Because of such flexible pathways of fetal development, what is called "a premature birth" or "being born before the time" is, paradoxically, *not* expressible in terms of fixed months or a particular gestational age. Instead, it indicates any birth happening before the necessary development of physical substance and life force has been completed. Premature babies are therefore described to be "not hard yet" (*mon atəka detä*) or "not filled yet" (*mon kolonde*). As the pace of their "filling" is contingent on the blood strength of the parents rather than on a set time interval, newborns can be considered premature at either five, six, seven, eight, or even nine months. That it is not *time* but the amount of *force* that determines the maturity or prematurity of babies was made clear to me in a discussion with Charlotte during a body-mapping session:

> *Charlotte*: If you give birth at five months, and if you have some chance, the child can live. For example, the husband of my aunt was born after five months of pregnancy. He is so old now that people call him "papa." When he quarrels with his wife, he says, "Even if I was born at five months, I am more solid than you are. I can hit you and you will fall." And it is true: he is very strong!
>
> *Me:* How do you call these children who are born at five months and continue to live?
>
> *Charlotte*: We call them mon kolonde. So the child is not born in its entirety. Like when you fetch water in a bucket that you haven't completely filled. You can use the same word *kolonde* to say that the bucket is not entirely full of water.

Me: From which moment can you call a child kolonde?

Charlotte: From five months. But even at six months it can be mon kolonde. And they often tell me that even some children of seven months can be mon kolonde. And still, many women give birth at six months. I know a girl who always gives birth at six months. And all these children are normal and alive.

Charlotte's first example is insightful: the man's assurance that he is solid and strong is not only a reaction to the perception that children born at five months are "unfilled" and lacking in force, but it also proves that whether a premature baby continues to live or not depends exactly on this amount of physical force present at birth. Of all babies born at a certain gestational age, some may live while others die. Some have reached their full maturity while others are "born before their time" with too small an amount of force to ensure survival. Although Charlotte reciprocates my time-based questions with time-inspired answers, the inconsistency of her definition of mon kolonde shows that questions about preset periods are in fact not the appropriate ones to ask.[8] The irrelevance of fixed time frames as a basis of prematurity and viability was again stressed by Peggy, who carried a pregnancy of eight months and wondered why her baby waited so long to initiate childbirth. Since she had always given birth around seven or eight months, she assured me that her child must already be "growing old" in her belly now. She contemplated:

In the hospital they often say that a child is premature from seven months onward. But that is not necessarily the case. There was a woman here who always gave birth after seven months. And all her children were born normal and alive. Well, and in the hospital, they say that at eight months, the child is dysmature [dysmaturé]. So that means that he can already be born, he has already everything, but certain organs or functions are not totally developed. But I don't understand. How can that be? Certainly not all children are dysmature at eight months, since others can be born normally at seven months already.

I asked Peggy how one could know whether a baby born at seven months would be normal or premature. Her answer was that those who are not fully "filled with force" cry less loudly than babies who were born "normally" after seven months, and that they lack a sucking reflex as their jaws are still under-developed and tender.

These Gbigbil conceptions of vital force are at odds with predefined bio-medical categories of viability, which take gestational time or birth weight as its exact, independent, and measurable indicators. Medical specialists have increasingly come to phrase the uncertain survival chances of premature children in terms of calculated risk assessments that downplay physical strength and bodily fitness in favor of measurable time and weight (Downe and Dykes 2009; Einarsdóttir 2009). In their paradigm, lack of force is only a *consequence* of a premature birth at a certain, fixed, point in time rather than a *contingent constituent* of prematurity—as Gbigbil embryology has it (see also van der Sijpt 2010, 2013).

Since Gbigbil people determine viability not by linear time or a particular weight, but rather by the amount of life force, which in turn depends on particular social circumstances and on the physical attributes of related others, I propose to speak about "contingent viability." I hereby draw on Bledsoe's notion of "contingent lives" (2002). Bledsoe shows how in rural Gambia, ageing is perceived to be a result of the traumas encountered over the course of personal history rather than an effect of the passing of linear time. She argues that "the whims of fortune to which our lives are subjected produce immense unevenness in the pace and character of bodily transformation, both within the span of our own lives and from one person to another" (22–23). It is exactly this conditional unevenness in the pace of physical transformation that also underlies notions of viability and maturity of newborns in Asung. Gbigbil ideas of "contingent viability" defy the linear and teleological assumptions informing Western visions of embryological trajectories; they show that the beginnings and endings of life are *contingent* local concepts, which are never stable or self-evident (Kaufman and Morgan 2005).

Indeed, Gbigbil views on embryology allow for different interpretations of what a pregnancy contains at particular moments, and when human life and a "soul" enter. Some women pointed to the commencement of human, God-given life right at the moment of conception; others considered life to evolve with human forms after three, four, or five months; and still others claimed that human life is proved only outside the uterus, when a child is born alive and with enough force. Conceptions about the entrance of a "soul" into a child were similarly diverse. Some suspected this to happen at the moment of quickening, others reasoned that it must be at the moment of the first cry upon birth, and yet others assumed only a gradual development of personhood over the life course.

The following chapters will illuminate how this multiplicity of interpretations allows for flexible accounts of not only what is formed during a pregnancy, but also what is lost during its interruption. For now, it suffices to conclude that the beginning of the lives of Gbigbil babies is a contingent and conditional matter. This is even more so because, apart from its contingency on parental physical attributes, fetal development depends on the behavior of mothers and others in the social and supernatural worlds.

Pregnancy Sorrows and Secrets

Reproduction is a contested issue in Asung. It is a source of hostility or alliance between two lineages, a source of security or insecurity in the fragile relationships between two partners, and a source of struggle between co-wives or other female competitors. In this context, reproduction is constantly surveyed and possibly influenced by others—with good or bad intentions. Before, during, and after their pregnancies, Gbigbil women are constantly being watched and are watching other women themselves. When bathing together in a river after working in their fields, for instance, women easily notice who is missing (which occurs during menstruation, since women do not bathe in public during their periods) and who has been washing herself there for too long without interruption (indicating a potential pregnancy). Within households, women often share sanitary towels and can thus keep track of each other's reproductive happenings. It is in this way that missed periods may be suspected by sisters or sisters-in-law. It happened to my informant Charlotte. Her older sister had not only noticed that she didn't use sanitary towels anymore but also knew the exact dates of her last menstruation and sexual intercourse; as a result, she knew that her younger sister was pregnant even before Charlotte realized it herself.

Given this public scrutiny, women are careful in disposing of their menstrual blood. Many of them prefer to wear loincloths or torn pieces of their babies' diapers (*niinda mekil*), which they can wash at the end of the day and reuse afterward. Others do wear disposable sanitary towels but carefully burn them or throw them away in a river or in the deep hole of the lavatory, so that nobody with evil thoughts could get ahold of their blood. Menstrual blood is thought to be a powerful substitute for one's fertility when used in local remedies (*bile*). Malevolent others may try to "steal" a woman's blood and negatively affect her childbearing capacities with it.

But menstrual blood also plays an important role in women's own attempts to influence their fertility. By symbolically "blocking" their flow of menstruation—through burying menstrual blood that is put in a bottle, stuffed in a snail shell, or attached to a needle—Gbigbil women aim to temporarily or definitively stop their childbearing. Such local contraceptive practices are widespread, applied during various stages of the reproductive trajectory, only to be discontinued or interrupted afterward, or to be combined with, or replaced by, the use of modern contraception. Western birth control methods are resorted to just as flexibly and temporarily (cf. Bledsoe 2002; Bledsoe, Banja, and Hill 1998) but are slightly less popular owing to their price, as well as to the notion that especially female-controlled methods such as pills and injections would permanently impair one's fertility. Most women like having the possibility to "block" or "unblock" their flow of fertile blood in line with their predicaments and their life projects at various points in time. As we will see, they may use indigenous methods, modern contraceptives, but also abortions to this end.

Despite the constant surveillance of menstrual cycles by women themselves and by others, it is often not the absence of blood that first signals "the entrance of a pregnancy" to them. Many women assert that they recognize a pregnancy even before they determine a missed period. They mention inner bodily transformations such as a quicker heartbeat and an increased weight and temperature, as well as distorted bodily functions, such as intense fatigue, headache, nauseas, unusual cravings for food, or "des petites maladies" (little illnesses). Outer appearances also change: the complexion becomes lighter and facial appearance more shining, the navel points out, nipples blacken, and a black line appears from the pubic area up to the navel or higher. Based on these various visible signs, the experienced eye will easily remark that a woman "has become more beautiful" and that "there has to be something." Gbigbil mamas do not refrain from warning girls on the street that they "have eaten bananas" (*obəng dyĩ ayola*), "have collected something" (*obəng vubele*), "have a baggage" (*onene bəppə*), "are well-positioned" (*osō itəlka*), or "are already women" (*osō munka*).[9]

Allusions to an early pregnancy remain always symbolic, though. To pronounce it by its proper name would expose a hidden, vulnerable state and thereby threaten the fragile zəng mon. Even though women know all too well what the metaphors of their mamas mean, they will do everything to hide and deny their pregnant state. Since an early pregnancy is considered to contain "only water water" or "a mass of blood," it is liable to destruction by jealous, infertile, or malicious witches, who are generally known to "suck people's blood." This threat to fertility comes most often—and somehow paradoxically—"from within," as witches are believed to operate in intimate circles, preferring to attack close relatives (Geschiere 2003). Therefore, a woman's family members and those of her husband (if she is married) should remain ignorant of the pregnancy for as long as possible. In some cases, however, Gbigbil women may inform their partners about the pregnancy in an early stage. This happens mostly in informal relationships in which commitments are loose and future projects uncertain. By announcing a pregnancy quickly, women attempt to convince their partners of their paternity and make them act more responsibly (see further Chapter 4). An early disclosure also offers women time to search for alternatives if their partners seem unwilling to commit; men's initial reactions are often crucial in deciding whether to keep a pregnancy, "give" it to someone else, or "evacuate" it altogether. Such cases aside, it is in a woman's interest to remain silent and deny every allusion to her changed appearance until zəng mon has transformed into a stronger and well-formed mon, and the pregnancy becomes more stable and secure.[10]

Only when the protruding abdomen becomes visible and acknowledged, does a pregnant woman acquire a status as such in the community. As denial of the pregnancy becomes unsustainable now, the initial secrecy and silence give way to public jokes, social interferences, and critical recommendations. Especially older women in her own family and those in her husband's compound will keep a watchful eye on the pregnant woman, for two reasons. First, surveillance is deemed necessary as ill-intended people may smell "the odors of pregnancy" or visually recognize the growing belly (even if it will be carefully hidden under a wide *kabba* dress that the pregnant woman will now start to wear). Not only could witches wish to "devour" the well-formed mon in their nightly gatherings, but those desiring a child themselves might mystically "steal" the fetus and place it in their own womb, after which the originally pregnant woman would see her belly disappear.

Second, control by others is warranted because the mother-to-be will be subjected to many prohibitions. As zəng mon has now more or less transformed into a human-like *mon* dependent on, affected by, and imitating its mother's deeds, prohibitions (*bikil*) pertain to the mother's moral behavior, daily activities, physical appearance, and food intake. For instance, the mother-child analogy prohibits laziness or standing still in the door opening since this would lead to a prolonged and difficult labor; wearing bracelets or necklaces would wrap the umbilical cord around the child's neck; eating porcupine would lead to the birth of a baby with a skin disease; talking about miscarriages would provoke one; and quarrelling with people would make *mon* refuse to be born quickly. Also the father-to-be encounters certain behavioral limitations.[11] While prescriptions are multiple and sometimes even contradictory, they all aim to preserve the well-being of mother and child, and to enhance a successful gestation and delivery.[12]

After six or seven months of gestation, a pregnant married woman often leaves her husband and in-laws to go and "wait for the delivery" (*atake bong abial*) with her own family. That this tradition holds particularly for the first pregnancy a woman carries for a man reflects the initial distrust between a (potential) daughter-in-law and her in-laws that has been outlined in the previous chapter. At home, women expect to get more rest, privacy, better care, and intimate knowledge of indigenous medicines enhancing a quick and safe delivery. These "remedies of the vagina" (*bile ndjol*) are inserted or evaporated into the vagina, "vaccinated" in the lower back or waist, carried in underwear or in cords around the hips, or introduced into the rectum through an enema—all with the aim of enlarging the pelvic opening.[13] Since pregnant women are not supposed to have sexual intercourse during this last phase of pregnancy, these remedies are deemed essential to "keep the route open" and help *mon* to quickly find its way out at the moment of delivery.

The intimate sociality of preparation for labor stands in sharp contrast with the ideal of solitary management of childbirth itself. Many older women proudly relate how in earlier days, women were so brave as to give birth alone in the bush. They proved their womanhood by not showing the labor pains they suffered—as self-mastery, resilience, and endurance are appreciated indicators of women's dignity in this region (cf. Johnson-Hanks 2006)—by silently withdrawing themselves behind the huts, and by giving birth all alone in the fields or on the coffee plantation.[14] Although I did not hear of any solitary births actually happening while I was in the field, it remained a norm that even the youngest women mentioned—either because older women confronted them with it or because they themselves liked the idea. Sophie, a twenty-seven-year-old woman, related the experience of the birth of her fourth daughter as follows:

> My younger sister gave birth to her first daughter all alone, behind the house. She called out, "Come-oh, come-oh!" People found that the child was already born. Eke! I also wanted to try this. So I did not tell anybody about my labor pains. I was there, I sat, I just endured and endured while the pain persisted. Ha! You must be very courageous, huh? I didn't succeed. At nine o'clock in the evening, the child said, "You're lying, I want to get out now." I want to sit, no. I want to stand up, no. My mother and sisters ask me what's wrong. I ask them, "Ever since I have been talking with you, haven't you noticed anything?" Everybody was so surprised to know I had been in labor all the time! They ran to call my older sister and mama Adèle [a traditional midwife]. I pushed once and I already had my child in my arms. The next morning everybody was surprised. Nobody had known and I had endured a lot all alone.

The ideal of showing independence, force, and endurance notwithstanding, most deliveries eventually happen in the company of some female relatives. They install themselves in the kitchen or in a secluded room in the house, where the entrance of men and children is strictly prohibited. As soon as the delivery is near, a mother or sister will run to call a traditional midwife (*munka mebyala*) for assistance. These "midwives" are often older women in the family, who have gathered experience throughout and after their own childbearing years.[15] The parturient is installed on the floor and supported by a woman—her mother or sister—sitting behind her with open legs and holding her arms. The birth attendant will wait in between the parturient's legs to "catch the baby" (see also Figure 2) and cut the umbilical cord with a razor blade.

Whether they give birth alone or in the company of others, women recognize that childbearing always involves risks. The fears that exist around birth were made most clear to me during Marianne's labor. I had been called to assist this childbirth at ten o'clock in the evening, when the village was already dark and quiet. Angélique, Marianne's sister, had come to my room and had whispered, " It has started." Armed with a coat and my torch, I had accompanied her, in silence, to her paternal home at the other side of the village. I had found Marianne sitting on the earthen floor of the living room, surrounded by her mother and her mother's co-wife.

We waited for a whole night, but Marianne's labor did not show any signs of progress. Angélique was constantly administering remedies to her sister. First, Marianne had to drink a mixture of garlic, onion, and ginger, which was thought to "pick" the child; then, she had to rectally insert rasped coco yam (*mekappa*), which was believed to "scratch" the child; after this, another enema of small peppers (*sonde*) and soap (*soppo*) was administered to "heat" the child; honey was constantly near to "energize" the child; every now and then, Marianne's belly was gently tapped by her mother to "awaken" the child; and finally, when we all wanted to sleep, Marianne was instructed to walk around in the dark room and jump if she would cease to feel fetal movement. With all this, the women hoped to accelerate labor and have Marianne deliver before the morning would arrive and other villagers would discover her absence from Asung's public life.

Unfortunately, the remedies had no effect. The next day we forced ourselves outside to keep up appearances; we sat, laughed, and worked in the courtyard, pretending nothing was going on inside. But Marianne was left alone in painful labor that did not advance. The second night did not bring any improvements either. Angélique and her mother anxiously discussed whether it would be more dangerous to stay at home or to go to the village health center a few hundred meters away. While her mother proposed to stay home, Angélique insisted on resorting to the hospital. Only in the early morning of the second day, just before sunrise, did her mother hesitantly allow us to take Marianne to the doctor. Again, as we had two days before, Angélique and I walked through the village in silence and darkness—now accompanied by Marianne, who was not supposed to be seen by any outsiders. Only half a day later Marianne gave birth to a daughter. Although visibly relieved and happy, her mother couldn't refrain from grumbling that nowadays young women don't know how to endure labor pains in silence and secrecy—thereby exposing themselves to needless risks. Other women nodded affirmatively, and Marianne did what she had been expected to do some days before: she bent her head and kept silent.

The fears that arose around Marianne's delivery were multiple. The longer labor lasted, the more they intensified. In the first place, an *accouchement difficile* (*abial yaka*) like Marianne's is physically damaging and exhausting. Dramatically diminishing one's repository of "life force" and blood, it can eventually be fatal. More than once during Marianne's prolonged labor, her mother and sister told me that "l'accouchement, c'est la mort" (birth is death). When we silently left Marianne alone in the house and installed ourselves in the courtyard, Marianne's mother looked approvingly at the black clothes that I happened to wear. She whispered that I did well to wear these clothes today, "because we are all mourning." This association between birth and death is not far-fetched; many women in this region die during pregnancy and childbirth. Although it is difficult to obtain reliable maternal mortality figures at the local level, the national estimate of 782 deaths per 100,000 births (DHS 2011), as well as the many stories in the field about women dying because of labor complications, and the several "near miss" cases that I witnessed myself are indicative of the situation.

Second, lingering labor is also feared to attract social attention. The longer labor lasts, the more people might become aware of it. Among them may be witches, jealous co-wives, or people with a "bad heart" who might try to "block" or "attach" the delivery (*akomma abial*) through symbolic or occult actions. In order to prevent the pregnancy from "descending," they might suspend attributes symbolizing the parturient's fertility—for instance, her underwear or the stone used for grinding condiments (*akok*).[16] Unless the ill-wishers undo this action, the child will not "find its way out" and could die in utero. It is the fear of such interventions that inspires women's preference to keep silent during labor pains and to give birth all alone, far away from people with bad hearts and bad intentions. It also explains why the labor of women like Marianne, who *do* give birth in the company of others, is surrounded by silence and whispering, and does not involve public appearances unless the darkness of the night has closed the eyes of other villagers.

At the same time, labor complications may turn suspicious eyes toward the parturient herself. As mentioned earlier, problems may be caused by a woman having had sexual intercourse with men other than the father of the child (*ibamba*). Joséphine, who gave birth for the first time when she was twenty-three years old, almost cried when she told me that some women had come to the hospital—where she had been transported after prolonged labor—to ask her to confess her sexual activities so that the child could be born. Another young woman, Daniëlle, who *did* "mix" her pregnancy, recalled that she barely managed to escape the embarrassing situation during labor in which she would have had to cite the names of all the men she had slept with. Thanks to the remedies her mother had given to her—and on which she had to pee daily while pronouncing the name of the genitor—her delivery had gone smoothly and had not raised any eyebrows. Next to transgressing sexual taboos, women may be accused of having ignored other behavioral prescriptions during pregnancy, or of having neglected the application of the "remedies of the vagina."

In bad cases, the parturient may also be suspected of being a witch herself. Since the entity of witchcraft (ivū) is thought to be located in the belly, unborn babies might become the victim of its greediness during childbirth. The crab-like creature, which people often imagine the devastating power to be, might keep a hold on mon and refuse to let it go. The only way to solve such complications is to confess to a traditional birth attendant to be a witch—something midwives claim to feel immediately during their first "toucher"; ivū, positioned in front of the child to prevent its descending, will "bite" midwives' fingers as soon as they insert them in a woman's vagina. Only after attaching certain remedies to the hand, which make the witchcraft "flee" upward in the belly and lose track of the child, can they help the child being born normally. In other cases, ivū is told to leave the vagina and vomit the child on the ground, while rendering the birthing woman in mortal danger as long as it remains outside of the uterus. Other women are noted to have given birth to an animal or an amorphous creature because of their ivū.

To conclude, birth is an ambiguous moment in the Gbigbil world. It is, like many of the preceding phases during pregnancy, contingent on both physical and supernatural forces. The uncertainty of its outcome leads to flexible interpretations of what is going on when things go otherwise than expected. It also leads to a range of practical and bodily interventions that help women manage the uncertainties and reduce their vulnerabilities.

Spiritual and physical vulnerabilities last until well into the postpartum period. Both the new mother (yal) and her newborn baby (tiaŋli mon) are therefore subjected to strict surveillance and prescriptions while staying with the woman's family members for some time. Yal is believed to be particularly weak in a physical sense; the flows of blood and breast milk—a derivative of blood—during delivery and the nursing period directly diminish her amount of blood and, by implication, force. There are several indigenous methods to restore blood and force levels in this period of intense depletion. First, daily massages (ba abum) are considered indispensable to heal the "wound of the placenta," evacuate all the "bad blood" from the uterus, and allow yal to regain strength.[17] Second, various indigenous remedies are believed to "clean the stomach" or replenish the blood reservoir with fresh and strong blood. Concoctions containing, for instance, papaya, eggs, milk, red wine, or mashed tomatoes—substances that resemble red blood or white milk—are widely consumed by women who are recovering after birth.

Although these remedies enable the body to replenish its blood reservoirs, they are only partial substitutes; one can never attain the previous level of force once a certain amount of blood has been lost. Or, in one informant's words, "It is only indirect. It doesn't give you blood like when you receive blood by transfusion. Compare it to vitamin pills: you can take them, but you will only gain weight some time afterward." It is in this sense that hospital injections are deemed most effective after deliveries. As needles enter the veins directly, they are thought to offer the quickest boost of vitamins, blood, and force. Ideally, many women prefer to visit the health center after childbirth; postpartum care will keep them energetic, strong, and well prepared for their next pregnancy, when they will be subjected to new physical and spiritual hazards. But how do they think about biomedical services *during* pregnancy? The discussions that evolved during Marianne's labor suggested a more complicated approach toward hospital attendance before birth. What are the perceived advantages and disadvantages of biomedical reproductive health care in this setting, where pregnancies are surrounded by many uncertainties and potential perils?

Pills, Pictures, and Prescriptions: A Continuum of Care

Asung's health center, like all Centres de Santé Intégré in Cameroon, is supposed to provide basic but comprehensive mother and child health care. The clinic offers antenatal services, including measurements and diagnostics of pregnancy parameters (blood, urine, temperature), and is endowed with a delivery room, a delivery table, and some rudimentary medicine needed for basic obstetric care and postpartum services. A total coverage of monthly antenatal consultations during the entire pregnancy costs approximately 1,500 CFA francs (around 2.25 euros); for normal hospital deliveries, women should reserve 5,000 CFA francs (around 7.50 euros). The missionary dispensary in the neighboring village of Kamandjom offers antenatal services at similar prices but does not facilitate deliveries. The bigger hospitals in Bélabo and Bertoua provide more advanced, yet more expensive, services—including ultrasounds and caesarean sections. Officially, women should prove that they have attended antenatal care before being admitted for a hospital delivery. In practice, however, it depends on the receiving doctor (if there is any) and on the circumstances in the clinic whether one is or is not received without a maternity booklet. Both doctors who were appointed to Asung's health center during my fieldwork—both coming from elsewhere in Cameroon—had had some form of obstetric training. They were sometimes assisted by a nurse from a neighboring village, and, if need arose, by a Gbigbil pharmacist with some obstetrical experience.

On a yearly basis, around a hundred pregnant women attend antenatal care in Asung's health center, and a handful come to give birth there as well.[18] Others visit medical establishments in the surrounding area—a situational choice that depends on the availability of personnel and medicines, personal connections, previous experiences, the financial capabilities of partner or relatives, the available means of transportation, and other contingencies. Overall, it is not uncommon to hear women say that they delivered some of their children at home and others in one (or more) of the health centers in the region; or that, before (some of) their home births, they sought prenatal care in one (or more) medical establishments. What is it that makes biomedical reproductive health care attractive to them?

First of all, the physicality of biomedical examinations corresponds with women's material pregnancy management. Despite their social and supernatural vulnerabilities, pregnancies in Asung are largely experienced and evaluated in terms of their materiality: pregnant women are constantly assessing their bodily fluids (vaginal secretions, water, blood, and blood balls), supervising their bellies (form, volume, color, temperature, and appearing lines), and interpreting physical symptoms (heartbeat, fatigue, headache, nausea, and cravings). Not surprisingly, the management of pregnancies is largely physical as well. Bellies are touched, liquids carefully observed, and numerous remedies "vaccinated" into the skin, introduced into the rectum, or inserted into the vagina. This materiality also pervades biomedical antenatal care: doctors' measurements and palpations of the belly, injections of substances into the veins, prescriptions of pills to be swallowed or vaginally inserted, and examinations of blood and urine add to a Gbigbil repertoire of pregnancy evaluations. Instead of being two opposed forms of pregnancy management, "indigenous" and biomedical interventions thus form a continuum of physical care—complementary rather than competitive.

Second, biomedical antenatal care offers visual facilities that give meaning and direction to women's embryological speculations. While many informants would answer my questions about female physiology and embryology with claims that "one cannot see what is in the belly" or that "our bellies are too deep to know," proponents of antenatal care stated that medical doctors "can see the condition of the belly" or "see how the child is positioned in the belly." In this setting, where normally only witches are believed to be able to "see" what is inside the uterus, visual biomedical technologies—especially ultrasounds—are credited with great powers.

The authority of these visual technologies almost paradoxically leads to a blind trust of women, characterized by ignorance of the exact process and mere acceptance of reported results. My informant Joséphine, for instance, expressed her surprise and indignation after her first ultrasound in the provincial hospital of Bertoua, during which she learned that she had been pregnant for seven instead of the assumed three months. Not only had she not expected the doctor to uncover her belly and "pour water over it"; she could also not understand that he needed only five minutes to "see" all the information and then simply sent her home again—a trip of several hours. That Joséphine could make no sense of the ultrasound was not surprising, as the doctor had turned the screen away from her and did not comment on what he saw. Nor was it surprising that she did not suspect the black picture in her maternity booklet to represent her fetus; it was simply not told to her. What Joséphine *had* understood was that her child "looked fine" and that she should now quickly urge her boyfriend to prepare the layette.[19]

A last attraction of biomedical supervision of pregnancies lies in its labor management. In this respect, women applaud hospital deliveries for two different, though opposed, reasons. Those fearing prolonged deliveries claim that hospital births are potentially quicker and safer owing to the presence of labor-inducing measures (such as oxytocin). Rather than experiment at home with "indigenous" remedies, of which the substance and required dose are often unknown, they prefer to ask a knowledgeable doctor for a quick and effective intervention. The injectable form of this intervention only reinforces its perceived effectiveness, as medicines that "enter the blood directly" are deemed more powerful. Labor inducement is not rare in Asung's health center; more than once I witnessed the doctor accelerating a woman's labor—though most often he did so to prevent the interruption of his own (travel) plans for the day.

While equally denouncing the obsession with quick deliveries "at home," other women recommend hospital deliveries exactly because of the noninterventionist approach. They applaud the fact that "doctors simply wait for the child and catch it" without many accelerating interventions. Particularly younger women with some degree of education or with urban boyfriends (who often insist on hospital deliveries), as well as older ones who have encountered problems in childbearing, are critical of giving birth "in the village." Their criticism is fed by the doctor who regularly scolds mamas and *matrônes* (traditional birth attendants) for keeping their daughters hidden "in the village" for too long and sending them to the hospital only in the case of complications—thus increasing the mortality and morbidity risks for both the parturient and her fetus. During the postpartum vaginal exam of a woman who had lost her baby in a dramatic delivery, the doctor's remarks were unambiguous:

> *Woman [screaming]*: Isn't it all right now, doctor? Oh, God! It hurts! Gently, please.
>
> *Doctor [inserting his entire forearm in the vagina]*: Is it your mother who made you deliver? It is pity that makes me take care of you now! But I tell you: the village is dangerous. The other day, they almost assassinated a pregnant girl there. The girl wanted to come to the health center. The old mamas told her not to go.
>
> *Sister of the woman*: She was alone; she couldn't act.
>
> *Doctor*: Even her husband wanted to come here.
>
> *Sister*: You know, we cannot contradict the old mamas. For the husband, it's his wife. It is not his daughter.
>
> *Doctor*: Yes, up to the level that the mamas did an episiotomy with their nails! That's organized assassination! You know, the child that has passed [i.e., died] could have accused his grandmothers in court. Just like this one here [i.e., the woman he is treating]. She stays in the village for her first delivery, whereas she has no passageway. I had already explained her problem to her! [He inserts a compress into her vagina and tells her to descend from the table. After offering her sister some gloves and bandages, he orders the women to go.]
>
> *Sister*: What should we do with these gloves? We don't use that in the village.
>
> *Doctor*: No, you can only cut with your nails instead! [To me:] They wanted to deliver at home, but it didn't work out, so they came here in the very last minute. Before that, the old mamas were in a hurry and scolded the girl that she should push. No wonder the child has died!

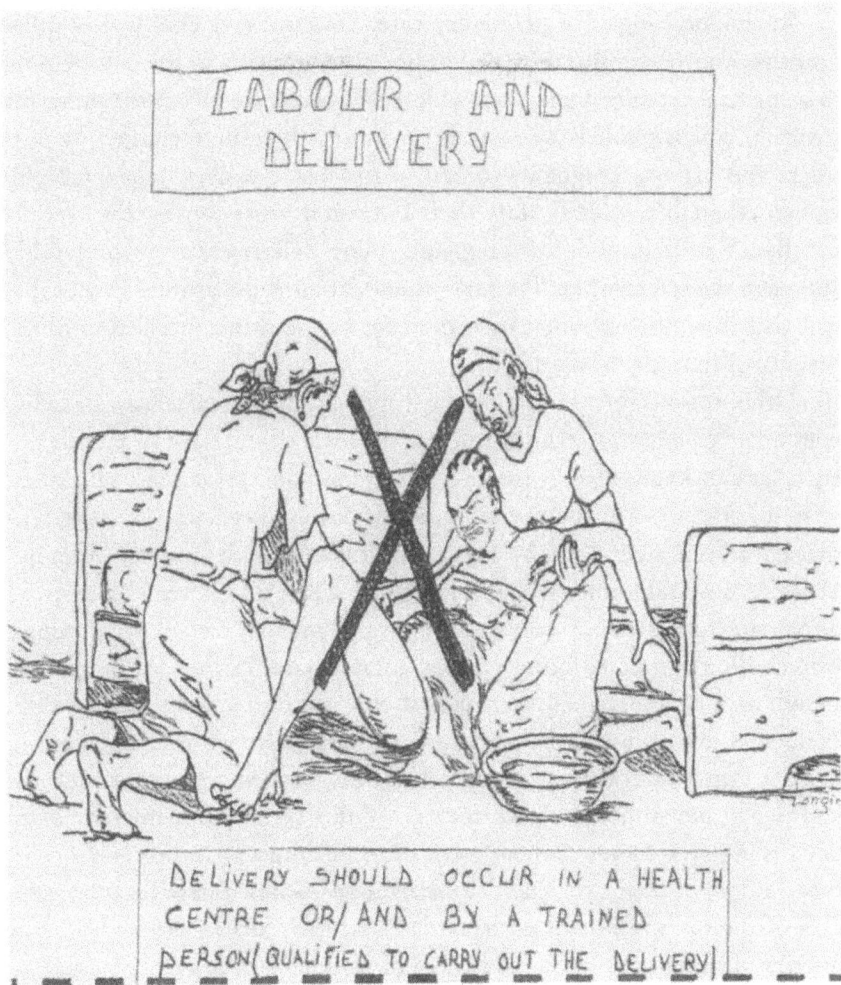

Figure 2. Poster warning against "risky" home deliveries. Source: Manual for the dissemination of information regarding the beneficial and harmful impacts of traditional practices affecting the reproductive health of the woman in Cameroon—distributed by Cameroon Medical Women's Association (1997).

The doctor's critical stance on home deliveries and the work of untrained birth attendants is reflected in many governmental and nongovernmental messages on maternal and child health in Cameroon. Advertisements like that in Figure 2, displaying "village" practices as harmful and risky, are well distributed over the country.

In the local logics of pregnancy care, however, it is exactly a hospital visit that may be considered risky for both the mother and the baby. Going to a medical establishment in a wide kabba dress (required for pregnant patients) equals publicizing one's pregnancy; it is easily remarked by outsiders and exposes pregnant women to the bad eyes of witches. Gbigbil women therefore seldom start their antenatal visits during the recommended first trimester of pregnancy. For deliveries, they preferably approach the center when it is dark—like Marianne did as well. Few people will visit them there, so that their presence can remain concealed until the first cry of the baby is expelled.

Other reasons for not visiting the dispensary for antenatal care or deliveries include embarrassment in front of the male doctor, lack of French fluency, lack of knowledge of the precise date of conception, lack of money, or simply the absence of any complications during pregnancy—motivations that have been mentioned by studies in different locales as well (Adetunji 1996; Asowa-Omorodion 1997; Beninguissé 2003; Chapman 2003; Olivier de Sardan et al. 2000). A delivery in a hospital requires certain preparations: women are required to bring medical utensils, and clothes for themselves as well as for the baby. Further, they should have attended antenatal care, as doctors may refuse to help parturients who arrive without a maternity booklet. Apart from these practical constraints, women may also contest the knowledge and authority of the doctors. With a history of many temporary doctors in mind—some of them good, some incompetent, others utterly corrupt, and all of them "outsiders" to the village—women have become skeptical of their promises and positions.[20] Particularly claims about the sex or number of fetuses, or about the safety of hospital births, are distrusted, as high-tech medical equipment is absent in the village center.

As local and biomedical logics of pregnancy care exist side by side in Asung—sometimes deemed complementary, sometimes deemed incompatible—young women constantly contrast medical recommendations with the daily "conseils" (advice) of their mamas. In 2008, a new doctor arrived in the village with a clear motivation to "get all pregnant women to the hospital." In one of his first educational sessions, he informed pregnant women about nutrition, hygiene, clothing, and antenatal care. While most attendants silently listened to his advice, some courageous ones articulated the discrepancies between his information and local prescriptions, in questions such as:

1. I will soon deliver my first child. The village mamas tell me that I shouldn't cut my nails, because the child would not be able to tear his placenta during labor. Is that correct? (In reaction to the advice of regularly clipping nails during pregnancy.)
2. Here in the village, they tell us that we shouldn't eat eggs, since the child will be born with dirt in his eyes. What to do? (In reaction to the recommendation of a protein-rich diet during pregnancy.)
3. Some people say we are not even allowed to "play," to "taste the ball," toward the end of a pregnancy. Is that true? (In reaction to the metaphorical advice of "playing football," i.e., having sexual intercourse, only intermittently during pregnancy.)

While the doctor dismissed these traditional prohibitions as *kongossa*—a popular word for gossip and false rumors—some youngsters rejected them either as means of older women to exert their power, or as pretexts for witches to attack. In the latter view, the prescriptions elders impose on them would be essentially meaningless; nonadherence would, however, provide an opportunity for witches to afflict the pregnant woman or "spoil" (*gâter*) her unborn child without being caught—since people would believe the situation to be caused by the transgression of the so-called pregnancy taboo (cf. Ministère de la Santé Publique Cameroun 1994).

This discussion shows how the contradictions between different pregnancy-related recommendations make many young women skeptical, both toward biomedical staff and toward their own grandmothers. At the same time, the multiplicity of prescriptions allows them to tactically deploy one interpretation or the other; depending on the situation, they can invoke "knowledge of the ancestors" and "knowledge of the whites" to justify their own practices. In this context, biomedical services add not only to the repertoire of concrete *care*, but also to the repertoire of *conceptions*. They thereby allow for different navigations and interpretations of pregnancy and childbirth by different women, and at different moments in time.

The tactical use of biomedical discourses and services in women's pregnancy navigations became clear to me when I went with my pregnant informant Charlotte for an antenatal check-up in an urban private clinic. Again, I was surprised about the lack of information she received while undergoing several examinations, and the lack of questions from her side; she assumed everything was "normal" as long as routine examinations were not interrupted or commented on. What seemed to interest her more was the amount of money her boyfriend would give her for the medicines and check-ups. When we met him afterward, she reported a much higher price for the prescribed medicines than what she had actually paid and untruthfully told him that the doctor had recommended an ultrasound in Bertoua. At that time, an ultrasound in the provincial hospital cost 7,000 CFA francs (around 10 euros). While many men deem an ultrasound necessary only in cases of serious reproductive problems, women assert or invent a need in order to claim, test, or use the feeling of responsibility of their partners—especially in fragile, informal relationships with relatively well-to-do "big fish" (see further Chapter 4). Charlotte succeeded; satisfied with the 5,000 CFA francs her boyfriend gave to her, she laughingly whispered to me that she had to make sure he would not ask for proof in her maternity booklet or insist on accompanying her to the clinic next time.

Not all women whisper, however. On the contrary, their tactics may be very well known by, or openly shared with, doctors and others. While I was having a chat with the doctor in Asung, Louise, a pregnant neighbor of the hospital who had never attended antenatal care, joined us on the wooden bench in front of the dispensary. When the doctor inquired about her well-being, the following conversation ensued:

> *Louise*: Today, I suffer more than on other days.
> *Doctor*: That's because you don't come to the hospital.
> *Louise*: I don't have money. It is hard for me to find even a hundred francs [.15 euros].
> *Doctor*: Don't you have cassava on your field that you can sell?
> *Louise*: I am planning to sell some this week in Dangi [neighboring village where her boyfriend lives]. I am searching money for the transport now. I will sell. Oh, *dokta*, can't you prescribe everything that you would like to prescribe in my maternity booklet? Everything! Even if I don't take it. But I will bring this to Dangi and tell my boyfriend, "This is what the doctor has prescribed." He will give me that money.

In the current absence of bride-price payments, some unwritten rules have developed that ensure a man's de facto right over his descendants as long as he acknowledges paternity and provides financially for mother and child. Paying for pregnancy-related care is an integral part of this process.

Gbigbil women like Louise may exploit this situation; they invent hospital visits to obtain money from their partners, even if that money is subsequently spent on completely different things. For them, biomedical care represents a starting point for alleviating relational and financial, rather than physical, risks that surround pregnancies in Asung.

It may be clear by now that pregnant Gbigbil women have ample room for secret maneuvers or discursive manipulations. This is so even if the reproductive process is, from the beginning to the end, inherently contingent on social and supernatural circumstances (such as the approval of God and the ancestors, the harmony within one's social relationships, or the goodwill of outsiders). Flexibly interpreting when conception happens, how a child develops, how a pregnancy can become endangered, and how it should be cared for, Gbigbil women navigate pragmatically through a complex fertility landscape. The following chapters will build on this insight as they explore what happens when pregnancies do *not* culminate in a live birth but are instead interrupted. How do women navigate such reproductive conjunctures, and how are the social, individual, and physical dynamics discussed in this chapter at play in the navigational process?

3

Rural Respect

All those baskets had hollowed out that sharp angle in her back like the notch in some tree stricken to death by the axe. The skin around that place had become as thick as an elephant's. "Is this my flesh and blood?" her mother had sobbed when Amalia still as flat as putty on the wall began to sulk about carrying the basket of provisions that they had made specially for her. "Who will want to marry a girl as frail as that?" she went on. "Who will ask for a girl in marriage when she can't even carry a basket?" [. . .] "The whole village is making fun of us," her mother told her. "Everyone says you aren't a woman . . . You can't even carry a basket . . . What will your husband eat?"

—Ferdinand Oyono, *The Old Man and the Medal* (1967: 55)

VERY EARLY ON A SUNNY MORNING, my adoptive mother mama Rosie rushes into my room with a pace that is quicker than her heavy body would seem to allow for.[1] Visibly wrought between the urge to deliver her message and the carefulness with which she wants to transmit it to me, she informs me that my friend Yvette has finally given birth, but that her situation is critical. I should really go and take a look. This message does not come as a surprise to me. Just a few days before, Yvette herself came to my room to discuss her fears about this delivery with me. Over the last few years, her reproductive experiences had become increasingly problematic. Four of her eight babies had died during or right after birth, and, as if this were not enough, her last catastrophic delivery had also left her with a debilitating fistula. Although she suspected her co-wife of having caused all this through witchcraft, her in-laws believed that it was Yvette who was "eating" their descendants in the occult world. Faced with increasing social and physical vulnerability, Yvette had tried hard to prevent another pregnancy but had failed. As a result, people had started to gossip, and her husband

and in-laws had declared themselves unwilling to take financial care of this pregnancy and its potential complications. Just a few days ago, here in my room, the pregnant Yvette strongly believed that her upcoming delivery would be a moment of life or death. I look into mama Rosie's eyes and realize that that moment has now arrived.

Fearful of what I will encounter, I rush to the maternity ward on the other side of the road. My fear proves to be justified; I find a naked Yvette lying in shock, with her arm pierced by an intravenous device provisionally attached to the window next to her, and her legs resting on a chair provisionally installed on the delivery table. She is surrounded by an enormous sea of blood and vomit. While the doctor tells me something about a retained placenta, anemic shock, and the imminence of death, I remain as silent as the two other women who witness this scene—one of whom I recognize to be Yvette's mother. I notice how silence also surrounds the package of towels on a table, which I know encloses the newborn baby. Hesitantly, I inquire about the condition of the child. The doctor affirms that although he was born with the umbilical cord wrapped around his neck, the little boy seems fine for now. But if nothing is done for his mother, she will be the one to lose her life.

As if protesting against this forecast of dying at the age of twenty-nine, Yvette slowly opens her eyes and tries to stretch out her arm to me as soon as she discovers my presence. I take this as a call for attention, closeness, and help; my initial silence suddenly turns into a sense of critical action. Though aware that my urge to help challenges the anthropological ideal of minimal intervention in the "natural course of things," I cannot but feel very implicated, and even strangely responsible, now. When I ask about the involvement of her husband and his family members, the doctor utters a scornful laughter. He explains that most of them have left for the fields today, as if nothing were happening. "They say there is no money anyway, and they don't care." His subsequent request for me to help out financially instead comes a bit as a surprise, but I show no hesitation. Though so far, I have avoided any financial involvement in my informants' reproductive lives and decisions, I realize that both time and Yvette's life are too precious to elaborately ponder over such ethical issues now. It is only with my money and the doctor's urgent directions that Yvette's husband and his relatives eventually go and search for appropriate medication in a nearby city. The short-term health improvement this induces in Yvette makes them decide to quickly take her home. Not long afterward, Yvette relapses, is transported to an urban medical center, and receives three blood transfusions before she regains consciousness.

After Yvette's return from the hospital, the fragile newborn boy—whom I named after my father when I was given the honor of choosing his name—refuses to drink his mother's breast milk. Wondering whether her milk is too poor after her heavy blood loss, or whether it is the effect of many different women having nursed the child during her stay in the hospital, Yvette goes to her paternal relatives in a neighboring village to search for indigenous treatment. When I visit her there, she happily shows me the black cords attached to the child's limbs, meant to increase his weight and force, as well as the concoctions that she drinks on a daily basis in order to "clean" her breast milk. Everything looks hopeful. However, on the day Yvette's husband Claude visits his wife and newborn son, my father's namesake dies. Yvette tells me, "The story of my son's death is a long story. No signs, no dreams. I played with him at 2 p.m., and one hour later, he was dead. I don't know anything. Is it a coincidence that my child died exactly when my husband paid me a visit? Is it my co-wife who sent my husband to kill the child?"

The exact cause of this incident is, however, much less a topic of discussion than its consequences are. The upheaval triggered by yet another child death leads both Yvette and her in-laws to reconsider the marriage between her and Claude. Yvette's priority now is to prevent any further catastrophic deliveries, and therefore to resort to reliable, modern contraceptives and to refuse intercourse as much as possible.[2] She even considers leaving the marriage; without a sexual relationship or emotional and financial support from her husband and in-laws, what is left to stay for? Her family-in-law, in turn, discusses what Yvette is still worth keeping for. Having spent a lot of money on her, without any visible results other than problems—with five of their descendants having died, with Yvette's current refusal to bear any more children, with her inability to engage in heavy physical activities, and with her continuous quarrels with her husband and co-wife—they decide that no bride-price payments should be transferred to Yvette's family. "They have concluded that my hospital costs cover my bride-price," Yvette relates in astonishment. It leaves her mother and paternal family members furious and the future of her marriage uncertain. More than once, I find Yvette throwing her kitchen utensils out of her mud-brick kitchen as a sign of determination to leave her husband—only to be discouraged by her sisters-in-law, who convince her that, after all, her own family cannot give the support and financial security she finds within this marriage.

Yvette knows they are right. There is almost no kin network from which she can seek assistance. As her mother had left her father when Yvette and her brother were still very young, Yvette spent most of her youth with her maternal grandmother, while her mother went back and forth between different marriages. This grandmother, who had also settled down with her own family after several failed marriages, was "a respected woman who worked like a man"; the enormous revenues gained from her work in the fields made her a safe haven for Yvette and all other children who had gathered around her. Her death left Yvette without any real source of support: the relationship with her own mother had always been problematic, her father had migrated to the other side of Cameroon, both parents had very few direct siblings to resort to, and her younger brother also died. Although her mother and paternal kin expressed their indignation now that they were told not to expect a bride-price, Yvette knows that it is unlikely that they will "come and take her out of marriage," as is often the case if bride-price is contested. Apart from feeling physically vulnerable, she realizes that she is socially isolated. Her position within her husband's family and the wider village is precarious, but she sees no other option than to stay.

Yvette's case may be extreme. She may have lost more children than many of her peers did, she may have felt more physically and socially vulnerable than other women with reproductive problems, and she may have encountered more explicit negative reactions from her in-laws and other villagers. Yet, it is exactly the extremity of her story that lays bare many of the (often hidden or latent) dynamics that evolve around reproductive problems in the village. Gbigbil women who had encountered reproductive interruptions, both before and after birth, often told me about similar struggles to assure their positions as wives and mothers. Their reproductive problems became associated with uncertain conjunctures in which their futures as respectable rural women were left hanging in the balance. Yvette's story thus illustrates common dynamics at play when fertility goes awry; its extremity just shows them more explicitly.[3]

This chapter will shed light on these dynamics. I explore why it is that reproductive interruptions endanger rural women's positions and aspirations, and how women like Yvette deal with this ambiguous situation. What options do they have to manage the complexities and contestations of the moment, and to ensure a respectful future in the village? In other words, how do rural Gbigbil women navigate the conjunctures that arise around their reproductive interruptions? To answer these questions, we have to understand what a life in the village looks like, and how it is imagined. As we will see, Gbigbil conceptions of the rural life course inform both the meanings of reproductive interruptions and the management of reproductive trajectories more generally. So let us continue where the previous chapter ended: at the vulnerable beginnings of the life course, once a Gbigbil baby is born.

The Vulnerable Beginnings of Life

As we have seen, Gbigbil people consider newborn babies (*tiaŋli mon*) to be extremely vulnerable. This fragility is first of all believed to be physical in nature. The gradual transformation of "water and blood" into a lizard-like creature and then into a "child" (mon) during pregnancy is only the start of what people see as a lifelong development of body substance and physical life force. Although newborn babies display all human shapes and body parts upon birth, they are considered very weak and "tender" (*tekaa*). Their delicate bodies are believed to be wet and to contain only "water water"—an expression that, like in the case of a beginning pregnancy, denotes the flaccid beginning of something that could become more firm later on. This body moisture results in a certain physical "looseness" denoted by the onomatopoeia *idəŋ dəŋ*, translated by one informant as "something slippery without bones to move with force." Indeed, the bodies of young babies still need to be filled with "hard bones" (*biveey*) and force (ngul); the process of "filling" the body that started during pregnancy continues after birth.

Maternal breast milk is deemed essential to this process: it offers "vitamins" and contributes to the development of bones and blood—and thus physical force—in babies. Without it, their bodies remain skinny, vulnerable, and exposed to death. Gbigbil mothers are therefore preoccupied with the amount and quality of their breast milk. Especially after heavy blood loss—which, because of a direct connection between body fluids, is believed to "deplete" or "spoil" maternal milk—they use various natural remedies to produce or purify their milk, and thereby enhance the "solidification" of their child.

These internal solidifications are often accompanied by a hardening of the outer skin, as mama Justine explained:

The skin of a newborn baby is still very tender (*iko nyol agin tekaa*). When the umbilical cord falls and the navel dries, the skin becomes a bit harder, and its color also changes. From three months onward, children can sit by themselves and are not carried around in towels anymore. From this time onward you can say *asó mon*: it is already a child. After that, the child will start to crawl, which again hardens his skin. He takes the form of a developing person now. As long as the child drinks his mother's milk we call him *aginne momon*: it is still a little child. But when he is weaned, it is really a mon. His skin also becomes like the skin of a real man.

Not surprisingly, a baby's skin receives special attention in many of the protective measures applied during infancy. In the first few days after delivery, for instance, a baby is not bathed in water for fear that its skin would become even softer. Instead, a newborn's body is rubbed with eggs and red powder (*bole*) to render it strong, healthy, and beautiful. Also, certain cords will be attached to the waist, ankles, and wrists in order to harden the skin, help the child gain weight, and protect him or her against typical "child illnesses" (*akón abongo*); these cords will be removed only when they are "filled with flesh and leave traces on the skin." Women like Yvette, who have been confronted with child death(s) before, are particularly eager to experiment with such treatments or to visit more experienced local healers for the physical care of their babies.

Next to this physical frailty, the beginning of life is characterized by spiritual vulnerability. Especially right after birth and in the first years of life, before they can talk with humans and reveal spiritual secrets, infants and small children are believed to remain in contact with the supernatural realm where they came from—called *ayong bekon* (the realm of the dead) or *ayong Zambe* (the realm of God). They communicate and play with the dead. One grandmother recounted to me how her two-year-old grandson had scared her while he was playing next to her in the fields. All of a sudden, he had started mentioning names and asked imaginary people to come and play with him. The boy had burst out in laughter and had become unresponsive to her calls. Only later, this grandmother admitted, did she understand that "he has people to play with, but it is only he who can see them; I can't." In the same vein, young children are knowledgeable of upcoming deaths in the village. Many mothers told me how their babies had cried unstoppably during the days and nights just before someone in their neighborhood died. Several remedies—such as black coal rubbed on babies' faces in order to ward off bad spirits and to have them "see only black darkness"—exist to make children less vulnerable to spiritual influences. Infants lose this connection with the supernatural world only gradually. The longer they live, the more their "human" life course takes over (cf. Gottlieb 2004; Molel Belika 2008).

Conceptualizations of the unfolding of that human life course are pervaded by an idea of predestination; the future of every person is somehow already "written" at the moment of birth. Children can be born to grow up as thieves or to become ministers—with the latter constituting a wish often expressed by Gbigbil mothers. Generally, the older a child gets, the more people see "the kind of person" he or she is to become. Once a child starts to play, talk, and listen to orders, his or her personhood, talents, and possible future paths are gradually felt and considered. But even before that time, destiny is at work. Indeed, it is in terms of spiritual predestination that the whims and woes of the fragile beginnings of life are often explained.

First, it can be exactly a person's *fate* to be born and to die immediately. Sometimes God wants his children back almost immediately after birth. "We don't know how many children God will send to us and how many he will take back" is an often-heard reason for bearing many children. God may have several reasons to reclaim his children. At the funeral of a seven-month-old boy, a priest wondered in his sermon whether any family members in the preceding four generations had committed some sin that resulted in "God saying that the child who shall be born will die." Something must have been done wrong in the family of the little boy, because "if God had wanted it, you would have discovered the illness before it got worse." A person's destiny is never purely individual but depends on the actions of social others, now and in the past.

Second, the opposite may also be true: a newborn child can be endowed with a great future, but it is exactly these wonderful prospects that are seen and destroyed by evil powers. Driven by their envy, witches may wish to destroy or spoil a child for whom a successful destination is "seen" lying ahead. They often attain this goal through transmitting their witchcraft to the newborn baby before the umbilical cord releases—a reason for mothers to hide their newborns inside the house and cover the umbilical cord with remedies enhancing desiccation. Witches may also send "a bad fate" (*le mauvais sort*) or other illnesses (biomedical or indigenous, general or specific "children's diseases") that prove fatal in young babies with little physical resistance or force.

Third, a child's spiritual connections might also interfere with the development of its beginning life course. Some toddlers are called by a dead relative. This was exactly what people had feared would happen to the two-year-old daughter of Michelline, a young woman who had died with an ectopic pregnancy. Since the child had been crying unstoppably at the funeral, everybody was convinced that Michelline was still lingering around to take her much-beloved daughter with her. A funeral attendant told me that they would soon have to treat the girl with indigenous remedies to make Michelline retreat. If not, the child could easily die—just like the attendant's own baby boy had, when he followed her deceased husband in a similar way.

Other babies might choose by themselves to "come to show their face only" or to "come in order to return immediately." Babies may have several reasons to "leave" immediately after birth: some foresee their own predestined, meager future and "flee" back to their safe haven; others might be angry or insulted about something people said about them—which is an important reason to be wary of excessive praising of newborn babies; and yet others come just to "tease" their parents from time to time. Such babies come and go; they die and are born again. Clearly, the dominant idea of predestination does not preclude a certain agency of babies and young children (cf. Gottlieb 2004; Gupta 2002; Kaufman and Morgan 2005; Scheper-Hughes 1992).

Stories abound in the village about children having been born several times. In order to detect these deceitful children, people bury them with a clear physical mark—formerly a cut finger or toe, but nowadays just some incisions on the cheeks or elsewhere on the body—which can be easily traced on future babies. These "reborn" babies will be called "rotten" (*bebolɛ*), "earth" (*metɔkki*), or "hoe" (*ibakh*)—names that refer to the burial of the child who preceded them. Similar conceptions of rebirth are described by Einarsdóttir (2000), Gottlieb (2004), and Gupta (2002) for Guinea-Bissau, Ivory Coast, and other parts of the world respectively. In the East of Cameroon, these returning children are called "Mont Kupe," which is in fact a mountain in the South-West Province of the country—perceived as the place where spirits reside.[4] Mama Georgette explained the treatment of these children as follows:

> Mont Kupe children come to search for wealth here, because they are poor over there. The person is born naked, isn't it? But when he dies, he will be buried with cloths, coffins, and toys. All these things he takes with him to where he came from. Well, if we suspect children to come and go like this, we put marks on their faces. We don't want this kind of children here. You know, especially in our days, the layette might even cost 50,000 or 60,000 francs [75 or 90 euros]. You spend your money, and then you lose your child. That's painful. So when such a child has come back and gets ill, you should only send him bad words: "If you have come to search for my wealth, you will return just like how you came to earth: naked and without anything. Aka! If you cry or you are ill, I just throw you away! I don't care! Tomorrow or the day after, I will conceive another pregnancy. If you want to leave, go! It is not the first time that you come here. Look at the marks that they gave to you!" It is this kind of bad mouth that you must give to your child, so that he will not leave anymore.

Connected with invisible forces in multiple ways, infants are vulnerable beings who linger in a space between the realm of the living and the realm of the dead. What Mary Douglas (1966) theorized a long time ago about people without clear identifiable positions in society seems to hold for Gbigbil newborn children as well: their status is ambiguous, pervaded by both vulnerability and potential danger. This social volatility is exacerbated by their physical frailty and lack of force to resist bad influences.

Accounts of child deaths reflect this ambiguity. They are often contradictory, referring to both physical and spiritual liabilities at the same time. Yvette, for instance, explained the first child death she encountered as follows:

> My first son who died did not cry when he was born. Everybody told my husband, "Don't buy any clothes, this is not a baby, he will die." He made movements, but no sounds. He had no force. It is the jaundice I had in my belly that caused this. It tires the child out. Maybe that is why all my children die. Well, for this one, I can also say that they

killed him mystically. Because the delivery was very difficult. A lot of problems, a lot of blood that flowed. The midwife said that since the child was stuck, I must be a witch. That my witchcraft kept the child in my belly. Another midwife was called for help. They now started to say that it was my co-wife who had administered some remedies when she had suspected I was in labor. She had blocked my delivery. I was already very tired when I finally delivered the child, but the child lived. And for three weeks, the child lived well. But one night, when we were asleep, an owl [considered to be "the bird of witchcraft"] started to talk on top of the roof. The next morning, the child didn't drink my milk anymore. He lost a lot of weight and died. I don't know exactly what it was. I only know they killed him mystically.

The deaths of her other babies were also attributed to their "prematurity" and lack of force on the one hand, and to spiritual influences on the other. This amalgam of possible causations allowed Yvette to stress certain interpretations of loss over others. Depending on the situation, she would blame these losses on either the incomplete "filling with force" or the supernatural attacks of her co-wife—or both at the same time. Depending on the story, she would downplay or dramatize the reproductive interruption at hand. However, as we have seen, by the time Yvette lost her fifth child, the exact cause became less important than the consequences it would have for her further life course. To understand this shift of attention, and the consequences it has for reproductive navigation, we have to move beyond the beginnings of life and look at the development of the female life course instead.

Diminishing Force: Fields, Fire, and Fertility

Although still called *bongo tekaa* (tender children) until far into childhood, over time children are believed to gradually solidify with the intake of breast milk and, afterward, nutritious food. They can thus be increasingly exposed to external influences, heavy movements, and some occasional beating—deemed essential for a proper education. During this education, children are constantly evaluated on the basis of the force that they are able to display. While small children are encouraged to walk around with small cups or plates on their heads, from the age of six or seven "they should carry baggage and show how strong they are." Like in the epigraph at the beginning of this chapter, girls in Asung are challenged to prove their strength by carrying heavy yields on their heads after work in the fields. They often vigorously take up this task; more than once, I noticed some unease in mothers when their daughters insisted on carrying a package of field products or wood that almost equaled their own body weight. The physical vulnerability with which children start their lives thus gradually turns into a zealous display of *in*vulnerability, force, and resistance. Although much of this attitude is supposed to be the result of education, ultimately one's strength is grounded in one's blood, as mama Georgette made clear: "If you see a woman who walks tired-tired, with hanging arms and unable to lift her feet normally, you know that she is a lazy woman. She is so weak. But if you see a woman who acts like a man, yes! You know that she is very strong! Solid! It is the blood that is behind all this. So you can't force it to be strong if your blood is not strong. You can't. It's your creation. And you will always remain like that."

The demonstration of this force eventually allows Gbigbil men and women to attain respected adulthood. For men, this means that they should be capable of fulfilling heavy physical tasks, but also that they should have the ability to form a group of followers around them. As discussed in Chapter 1, the importance of male autonomy and authority has historical roots; combined with a notion of "force" it becomes an embodied constituent of respected manhood. One anthropological source notes that a young man in this region inaugurates his personal career when "he finds the force (ngul) to install himself on his own and found a new village" (Laburthe-Tolra 1981: 558). Another one states that it is through his control over others—especially wives—that a man "acquires sufficient personal "force" to enable him to become an autonomous focus of allegiance, that is, to found a domestic group of his own" (Houseman 1988: 54–55). Until today, similar perceptions are present in the village of Asung. Strong men are those who separate themselves from the family, build a compound, and lead a household with many wives and children. If unable to demonstrate this capacity, men are scornfully called "weak" or "men of nothing" (*mod asumba*).

Women, in turn, attain respect by thriving well in the conjugal context. Entering and maintaining a successful marriage is a central aspiration for most rural Gbigbil women. What Jane Guyer (1984: 74) described quite some time ago for the region reflects an attitude that is still dominant in contemporary Asung: "The whole cultural tradition favours being a wife over being a daughter or sister. All the incentives in the rural areas converge to encourage women to aspire to marriage and to remain married. Security of access to land, assurance of an inheritance of one's children and status among the women of the village depend on being married. At the village level, bride-wealth payment is still the means of acquiring these rights."

The success of a marriage hinges on women's fulfillment of conjugal duties that require physical strength: hard work in the fields, dedication to the household, and childbearing. An important criterion for men in selecting their wives concerns exactly their physical strength and solidity, which will allow them to take up these tasks. As married women in this region come from "outside"—another village or another lineage in the same village—and occupy an ambiguous position surrounded by suspicion and hostility, they have a clear interest in displaying these physical capacities. Such a display contributes to the rise of their status as strong, zealous, and committed daughters-in-law and reduces inherent marital tensions. Those who work hardest and produce most—both food and children—eventually become the most respected women of the village. Physical accomplishments thus become morally laden, determining who is considered a good woman and wife. They are central to a Gbigbil moral framework resting on what I call the "ethics of production and reproduction."[5]

That hard work is a key attribute to good womanhood and successful wifehood was made clear to me at the funeral of Adèle. Adèle was a young woman from Asung who had gone into a marriage in another village. She had died in the process of aborting a pregnancy out of anger over her husband's negligence. As bride-price payments had remained absent in this marriage, Adèle's family had insisted on burying their daughter in their own village. This served as a catalyst for the married women in Asung to ritually refuse this burial on "the ground on which we work so hard every day." In their symbolic revolt (*saŋba*), these "wives" of the village started to insult the "daughters" of the village, like Adèle. In an animated atmosphere, norms of womanhood and wifehood came to be discussed, imposed, and contested between older "outsiders" (the "wives" who married into the village) and younger "insiders" (the unmarried "daughters" of Asung):

> *Wife 1*: The daughters of this village don't have any plantations of cocoyam, nor of cassava. They can only pick leaves to sell at the market [i.e., do very light work].

> *Wife 2*: But they don't stay in their marriage for a long time, do they? Their husbands refuse them, because they can only pick leaves. You, daughters of Asung, are refused everywhere.
>
> *Wife 3*: It is laziness that hampers you all. You can only think of picking leaves, going to the market, and doing *niangá* [making yourself beautiful].
>
> *Daughter*: Lazy?! Look at you, how skinny you are [to Wife 3].
>
> *Wife 2*: You insult her because she is skinny?
>
> *Daughter*: Well, is she strong then? She has no force.
>
> *Wife 3*: Even if I sit down, I am busy preparing, selling stuff, or I have people who work for me on my fields. But you, daughters of Asung, you tend to sell everything. You forget that you have a family to feed. Whereas we, wives of Asung, we are "those who *can*," not "those who *want to*."

By relating marital success to a persistent work ethos, the wives reiterated the dominant moral framework. The daughter's playful insult, however, points to the other side of the story. While the display of force might provide women and wives with social status, it also depletes the total amount of strength the body possesses. The force that is accumulated over the years through nutritious food intake will gradually diminish and induce a process of ageing and degeneration. Mama Rosie, who bore only one son and remained subsequently infertile, summed up several factors of depletion:

> Your force diminishes in the first place because of all the work: working in the fields, in the sun, carrying heavy baggage, searching for wood, preparing meals. You become worn-out. But also all illnesses that are in your body diminish your force. You don't eat well anymore; your mouth has become bitter. Also when you give birth, you lose your force. Your body diminishes, and you lose weight. And then you continue to nurse your baby for two years. After weaning the child, you carry another pregnancy. You lose your force in all these cases. Your blood becomes weak. So there is a visible difference between one woman who has borne one child in her life and a second one who gave birth a lot. The first woman is able-bodied; the second woman is tired, has lost a lot of weight, and has become dry-dry. She has no force left.

Because of the link between force and blood, a body's reservoir of ngul is directly depleted through flows of blood and breast milk during delivery and nursing. But also heavy work on the fields and illnesses "finish the body," as does the fire on which meals are prepared. A market woman told me that "the blood of women who prepare beignets every day will diminish because of the heat of the fire. Our fire is brutal. It makes the blood black and hot, and it diminishes its amount."

Apart from the *symbolic* connections between women's agricultural, culinary, and childbearing pursuits in marriage (also noted by Feldman-Savelsberg 1996; Goheen 1993; Houseman 1988; Johnson-Hanks 2007; Laburthe-Tolra 1981; and Notermans 1999), there is thus a clear *physical* component that underlies these tasks: fields, fire, and fertility all take their tolls on the body. Living up to the ethics of production and reproduction may contribute to one's social status, but it also renders the body old and worn-out. Thus, over time, bodies become as weak and low in force as those of young children; they are, just like newborn bodies, denoted by the Gbigbil word *tekaa* (weak). Yet, while the bodies of babies are perceived to be wet and tender, ready to begin a process of hardening and solidification, at the end of life the skin is thought to have become "hard" and "dried up" (*kotaa*)— reflecting a body devoid of blood and force.

This degeneration of the skin can be combated only by intense maintenance (*entretien*) of the body surfaces. Body lotions are deemed the best remedies in this respect. Many were the women who, after praising my white skin for its tenderness, would ask me for the creams and ointments they assumed I must have been using. They repeatedly regretted their lack of body lotions and the unwillingness of their husbands to provide them with these products. In fact, with the depletion of life force and ageing of the body reinforced by women's duties in marriage, the complaints about neglected skin formed an idiom to express both one's commitment to marriage obligations and one's frustration about not getting anything in return from the husband. Conflicts about body lotions are therefore at the center of negotiations of conjugal responsibilities. In her reaction to Yvette's threats to leave her marriage out of anger over Claude's negligence, for instance, the relatively young Frédérique lamented, "That's what always happens to me as well! I bore a lot of children but have never been maintained after deliveries. No hospital care, no injections, no pills. My husband doesn't give me money and doesn't care. He even neglects giving me oils and creams! That's why you see my body as worn-out as you see it now."

The process of physical degeneration that happens over the Gbigbil life course is thus a contingent one—more dependent on one's lifestyle and on encountered incidents than on one's exact age. Those who work hard to fulfill the ethics of production and reproduction lose their force quicker and grow old faster than those who do not. Those who are not properly "maintained" in the process do so too. As a result, women who seem relatively young in terms of age may call themselves "weak" and "old" as if they had reached the end of their life course. Similar conceptions have been described for Gambian women by Caroline Bledsoe, who argues that the "pace and character of senescence are contingent on cumulative wearing events such as reproduction that erode life's sustaining forces, with harsh experiences causing disproportionate loss" (2002: 322).

Indeed, while a certain degeneration over the female life course is acknowledged and expected, extreme deliveries and pregnancy interruptions, such as the ones Yvette encountered, upset this anticipated trajectory. Options to obtain respectable womanhood are affected as a result. Such reproductive happenings, then, are conjunctures that potentially alter both the physical and the social pathway of life. Not surprisingly, the meanings and management of these conjunctures are informed by the Gbigbil conceptions of the life course that were outlined above. The rest of the chapter will illustrate this point. I will explore both the interpretations and the implications of reproductive interruptions and, in the process, shed light on the reproductive navigation of Gbigbil women in this rural setting.

Falling Pregnancies and Forceless Babies

When talking about reproductive interruptions, Gbigbil people distinguish between the interruption of a *pregnancy* (abum), where no clear human being is formed, and the loss of a *child* (mon), presenting human forms. The previous chapter described how the first months of a pregnancy are considered "void" on the inside. At most, people speak about "water water," "blood," or a lizard-like creature. A loss that happens at this moment is usually called *abum ia song*. In my efforts to unravel the meaning of the verb *song*, I encountered an insightful metaphor given by a male Gbigbil student:

Song can be comprehended as the movement of a falling cup. Imagine that the cup contains something inside—water, for instance. At the moment it falls, it turns upside down and the water flows. You can then say, "kop ia me song a mo" [the cup falls out of my hand]. This is similar to what can happen to a pregnancy. In fact, conception of a pregnancy resembles the idea of the cup. A beginning pregnancy contains water water. Only by turning it upside down can the water flow. So "abum ia song" indicates this capsizing movement of a pregnancy in which the child has not yet been formed.

Tellingly, you do not "lose" a pregnancy: your pregnancy can be "falling" (*abum ia song*), "coming out" (*abum ia so*), or "leaving" (*abum ia vawa*). My informant Sophie explained the specific workings of this "fall," again metaphorically, through the expression *abum ia bugiye*:

We use the word *bugiye* when you break something partially. If you break a pen, for instance, the inner part remains, the outer part falls down. The same happens during pregnancy. The small fetus that develops inside is surrounded by blood. So when it does bugiye, this surrounding blood breaks off and falls down. The inside remains but cannot stay long for lack of blood and will come out afterward. So when the blood flows and the fetus is still inside, we can say, "mekil me bugiye abum" (the blood breaks down from my womb/pregnancy).

Sophie specifies that this process can take place only when the developing fetus is still surrounded by its constituting blood—which reminds us of the distinction between zəng mon, a nonhuman embryo developing inside a ball of blood, and mon, a fetus with distinctive human forms, as described in the previous chapter.

Once the watery substance of zəng mon has given way to something more firm and human-like (mon), the pregnancy itself is also said to be "hard" (*abum iso detaa*). It can no longer fall or break. Denotations of pregnancy interruption change accordingly: the expulsion of the fetus is now phrased in terms of the delivery of a dead child. Common expressions relate that "the child has passed" (*mon ia nul*), "the child is dead in the belly" (*mon ia wa abum*), "she has given birth to a child who is dead" (*abiali mon ia wa*), or simply "the child has died" (*mon awali*). Most of these expressions are also used to denote perinatal and neonatal losses or even infant and child deaths. Indeed, while such biomedical terms are based on strict temporal divisions (and on notions of viability, which are often also time based), for Gbigbil people it is not so much time in itself that underlies the various forms of loss and viability of children.

Although my informants distinguish the interruption of a pregnancy containing zəng mon from the loss of a visibly human creature called mon, the exact dividing line between the two is fluid and contested. Since zəng mon's development into mon hinges on the amount and quality of the blood—and therefore, force—of both parents, the difference between a "falling pregnancy" and a "passing child" cannot be traced to fixed linear time. Rather, what matters are the forms and force (zəng) mon displays upon expulsion. Only if human features are clearly discernible can the death of a "child" be talked about. As there is no conceptual distinction between a completely formed mon inside and a baby outside the uterus, whether its decease happens before, during, or after delivery is less relevant; in all cases, it concerns the loss of a formed child embodying the potential of life.[6]

Such fluid, ambiguous, and contested boundaries leave some room for women to strategically nominate what is actually lost—mere "blood" or a "baby." The same interruption may be defined as a "falling pregnancy" in one situation and as a "child death" in another. Again, we see how a certain ambiguity offers women the possibility to either downplay ("it was just blood") or dramatize ("a child was killed") their reproductive interruptions within the given circumstances and contestations. More than a fixed temporal framework, Gbigbil person-dependent and flexible embryology allows for person-dependent and flexible interpretations of reproductive interruptions (van der Sijpt 2010, 2013). It offers a rich terrain for negotiation of the beginnings and endings of human life (Kaufman and Morgan 2005).

Distinctions between types of interruption may become even more fuzzy under the veil of similarity invoked by the general notion of the "wasted womb." Whether talking about "falling pregnancies" or "child deaths" as the ones that Yvette experienced, Gbigbil people would often stretch their arms and show their empty hands, to convey the sense of emptiness that remains after *any* of these interruptions. No matter the specific moment and cause of an interruption, the possibility of having a living baby has been "wasted." "You are not left with anything, are you?" was the rhetorical question they posed while shrugging their shoulders. By talking about "wasted wombs," people stressed the fact that the meanings and effects of early and late reproductive interruptions may not be as different as the separate classifications suggest.[7] Instead, there are common consequences: all fertility interruptions make potential lives leave, and they all leave a woman's life with less potential.

This is certainly the case when we look at a woman's force potential. All "wasted wombs" imply a heavy toll on the body's reservoir of blood and ngul. The often-invoked expression "abortion is worse than childbirth"—with "abortion" denoting *any* reproductive interruption here—is explained exactly in terms of this excessive loss. The process of depletion is, however, different for early and late reproductive interruptions. In the case that a pregnancy "falls" in the initial phase of gestation, a lot of blood is shed: not only the blood that constitutes zəng mon, but also the surrounding blood that protects and nourishes the fetus. This abundance of blood loss *directly* causes an enormous diminution of a body's reservoir of force. Not surprisingly, women quickly resort to indigenous remedies that can prevent such a harmful situation. Biomedical help may also be sought, as injections are thought to be particularly effective in blocking the flow of blood. The registers of Asung's dispensary and two urban hospitals in the area revealed that the majority of the (few) cases of pregnancy interruption concerned mere *menaces*, rather than actual instances, of loss. If an interruption is considered inevitable, there are plenty of remedies "at home" to accelerate the process and, in this way, reduce the depletion of blood and force.[8]

Such depletion happens *indirectly* with difficult births in which the child to be born is weak or dead. A mother's loss of force is then inherently related to the decreased force of the baby. A child who is delivered "before his time" does not have the appropriate amount of force to initiate and manage childbirth by himself. Such a child becomes "tired" very quickly, drowns in the surrounding water, or simply dies from fatigue, and leaves it to his mother to finalize the delivery with her own force. This is what went wrong during Yvette's penultimate childbirth, which caused a fistula and a lot of trouble in her family-in-law:

> The child couldn't come out. So rather than that the child gave me the force to push, I had to push by myself, with my own force. It didn't work; I was already too tired. And so was my child. The midwives tore my

vagina all the way to the anus. Wanting to force my delivery, it is these village women who have killed my child. At the moment my child died in my belly, I lost my head. I screamed, "I only see darkness now. I don't see any people anymore." I was rolling in my own vomit. I don't know how they got to transport me to the hospital. It is only when the child had already come out there, and the doctors were sewing the wounds caused by these women, that I felt an enormous pain and opened my eyes. That's when I saw my dead baby lying on the table.

In cases where the child has already died in utero, this effect is even aggravated; with no incentive from the dead fetus at all, the delivery demands an enormous amount of a mother's force. It happened to Jeanette, who told me, "since the child was already dead, he could not get out by himself. So they had to push my belly and direct the child. At least, that's what people tell me, since I, I was already . . . I don't know. I was already tired, I could not even scream anymore. It was not even what they call fatigue. I was already dead."[9]

When both mother and child are at risk during childbirth, people will prefer to save the mother's life, and not the child's. The rationale underlying this moral choice—termed "life-boat ethics" by Hardin (1974)—was explained as follows by one informant: "In case of a difficult birth, there are many remedies that people can give you. And they can take you to the hospital. In order to evacuate the child. To protect the mother. Because we say here that when a mother and a baby fall into the water, you should always rescue the mother. You should leave the baby to die. Because you never know what would have become of the baby, whereas you know that the mother can still give birth to another one."[10] The encountered incident is considered just an interruption of a lifelong flow of fertility.

To enhance that expected flow of fertility after such critical reproductive interruptions, Gbigbil women resort to numerous treatments.[11] Even more than after normal childbirth, blood replenishment is deemed necessary now; women make abundant use of indigenous remedies and feel a more urgent need for biomedical injections in order to recover quickly. In this sense, my Gbigbil informants act like the Gambian women described by Caroline Bledsoe, for whom the length of fecund time is "a function of how well a woman takes care of her body" (2002: 323–24). Preoccupied with the maintenance of their blood levels, force reservoirs, and skin texture, Gbigbil women are as much "active shapers of their biological destinies" 325) as their

Gambian counterparts. Yet, biology cannot always be fully controlled, as Yvette's case showed all too clearly. Nor can the social world—the reactions of husbands, in-laws, family members, and villagers. Instead, reproductive interruptions, in reducing the both the force level and the social trust needed for establishing oneself as a successful woman and wife in this village, can pose considerable threats to the attainment of rural respect. How, then, do women like Yvette navigate these uncertainties? What options and obstructions do they encounter while trying to assure their present positions and their aspirations for the future?

Redefining Projects and Positions

When reproductive interruptions prevent women from fulfilling the "ethics of production and reproduction" that are so central to Gbigbil marriages, suspicions and accusations are prone to develop. Such negative reactions find their root in a *general* distrust toward daughters-in-law, who occupy ambiguous positions in the compounds of their husbands. Reproductive problems in particular exacerbate these latent tensions: since descendants are so much at stake for the patrilineage, but are only to be obtained through "outsiders" to the lineage, it is these outsiders who easily become blamed for the loss of (potential) children.

Suspicions often manifest themselves in witchcraft accusations. With the power of witchcraft (ivū) being situated in women's bellies, any reproductive problem—infertility, a pregnancy interruption, a problematic delivery, or the death of an infant—becomes easily explained in terms of that destructive force. As we have seen, women may strategically invoke particular interpretations of reproductive interruptions in order to downplay the event or direct the attention to *other* evil powers at play. Yet, for husbands and in-laws, fertility problems—especially if they are multiple, such as in Yvette's case[12]—induce doubt about a woman's status as a committed wife and a reliable mother; she might well be "eating" their descendants in the other world. Disgruntlement may increase if reproductive problems also prevent women from working in the fields and in the household. With a bride-price constituting *the* acknowledgment of a wife's status and contribution to the lineage, it is not surprising that the discussion often centers on this issue, rather than on the lost (potential) babies. While women would bring up their excessive bodily depletion as a justification for the transfer of a bride-price, it is exactly this depletion and its consequences (i.e., the loss of money, workforce, and descendants) that in-laws invoke for *not* paying it.

Both marital tensions and the absence of a bride-price are not uncommon in Asung, nor are they restricted to cases in which fertility has gone awry. The marital setting is generally characterized by flexibility; if frictions accumulate or bride-price negotiations fail, unions easily dissolve. Depending on their position in their families and families-in-law, their projects for the future, and the particularities of the reproductive conjuncture at hand, women can navigate a marital impasse in various ways. They may decide to stay and conceive again in order to show their goodwill and attenuate the tensions—hoping that the passage of time will turn their interrupted fertility into a nonevent. They may also go home for some rest and reflection. They may just leave their marriage altogether and search for another one. Or they may switch their life paths completely and try their luck in an urban setting.

Yvette deemed none of these options viable. Instead, she found an alternative way of managing the moment and plotting her pathway into the future. As we know now, each reproductive interruption constitutes a unique conjuncture in women's reproductive lives. The options and obstructions that such a conjuncture presents circumscribe the ways in which people can remedy the immediate situation and move toward an imagined future. Therefore, in order to understand the decisions and directions that Yvette took, we have to get back to the particular circumstances around the death of her last baby. How can we understand Yvette's navigation in terms of what was going on at that moment?

To begin with, Yvette had always occupied a rather particular position in Asung, which was not the home base of her father, nor the village of her mother's patrilineage, but the residence of her maternal grandmother. Although the return of a sister (and her children, who are called *mo kal*) to her brothers in case of a failed marriage is quite common and accepted in Asung, a situation in which the children of mo kal also settle in that family is rather unusual. Such children are likely to encounter even more hostility than their mothers (as mo kal) do in their maternal families.[13] Yvette had a similar ambiguous relationship with her (grand)mother's relatives. With the death of her grandmother, and later also of her brother, Yvette had lost the protective haven to which she could resort in case of marital problems. More than ever, Yvette had become an "outsider" in her own village; not only as a contested wife in marriage, but also as an unprotected child of mo kal in the neighborhood of her mother's maternal uncles. The quartier of her paternal family, in another village, was empty as a result of urban migration. The only uncle who had remained was openly critical of the departure of his brothers, as well as of the burden of the children they had left him with. The social distance he expressed toward Yvette was exacerbated by her physical distance; no substantive support was thus to be expected from the paternal side either. "Going home" for rest and relief was not really an option.

Apart from an impoverished kin network, Yvette also lacked other forms of capital that could have allowed her to explore alternative pathways into the future. Her first pregnancy, which she had conceived at the age of fourteen, had put an end to her then still starting secondary school career; the resulting lack of a proper education did not allow for formal training or employment that could help her move away from duties related to "field, fire, and fertility." To leave for a nearby city and search for an informal job or engage in petty trade would at least require some contacts facilitating housing and job orientation, which she did not really have. And her physical state, Yvette lamented, would not allow her to move away from the village either.

With no options beyond the village level, Yvette understood that, in order to stay there somehow respectfully, she would need to be married; "What can I do? It's the village." To resort to *another* marriage was, however, not an attractive option. Even *if* somebody would be willing to marry this "old woman with an old body"—as Yvette called herself—she would again have to fulfill the ethics of production and reproduction in order to establish herself as a wife and daughter-in-law. "It will be always the same thing: the man will first want to have intercourse in order to give me a pregnancy," she assured me. Since that scenario could possibly prove fatal, it was discarded as an unrealistic horizon.

With Claude, at least, she had agreed on the use of reliable birth control, and she was excused for her lesser productivity on her fields now that she had lost an enormous amount of life force for her family-in-law. To be married with a Bibakung man like Claude was not too bad either. Of all lineages in Asung, Bibakung was the most expanded and influential one: the few brick houses in the village were located in this particular neighborhood; the big plantations of the village were owned by Bibakung men; most of the elites who had successfully installed themselves in big cities or abroad were descendants of this lineage; and the village chief himself was too. Without a decent network of social support, Yvette was not unwilling to claim her dependency on this family. The Bibakung themselves felt less dependent on Yvette, though. Their relative status, the enormous number of descendants of Yvette's father-in-law (who had married four wives), and their knowledge of Yvette's vulnerable situation not only made them less reliant than many other families on their daughter-in-law's services but also gave them considerable room for manipulation.

So how did Yvette give meaning and direction to this uncertain marital situation? Even if she had a relatively disadvantaged social position and restricted room to maneuver, Yvette *did* rethink her marriage and her future, as well as the role of reproduction therein. Talking with me about her past and her envisaged trajectory, one year after her last delivery, she said:

> Look, all these deliveries turned me into an old woman. I was never maintained after birth like is usual in the village: massages with warm water, body lotions, hospital injections, and good food. These wash your stomach and skin and give you new force. But my husband even refuses to give money for soap or body lotion. He says I have eaten [*bouffé*] too much of his money already. And lack of maintenance makes women old. I lost a lot of blood and a lot of weight. It had to be recuperated all. With the blood I received in the hospital I had become very fat! But now I have to work hard again because these two years of illness have made my fields overgrown and unproductive; I have to recommence from zero. I have become like a child, although I spent so many years in marriage. Nothing is left, so I should work hard now. And automatically, I lose weight. I am still a little girl, but I am already old and skinny and my skin is ugly. Women of my age call me "old mama." You see?
>
> And since I don't even have any family to support me . . . On both paternal and maternal sides, there is nobody who can tell me, "Come, I will take care of you." If I had such a person, I would not even be here anymore. But now, if I would leave, where will I stay? No, I am in a marriage, and I will stay. And it is good to be married; if something happens to me now, people will search for him. Sleeping together or not, but I am with him. He will have to take care of me. But apart from that, here in the village, the marriages that people talk about, there is nothing in it except for suffering. It is only good if you produce children

and work hard on your field. Then, you are a person. Then, there is a marriage. So for me, it is really important to sacrifice myself to my field now. In order to ensure the future of those children who stayed. I stay in my marriage to take care of my children. I would also want to leave them with an inheritance. You see? I can't leave them behind like my mother did to us. I suffered as a child, I suffer here in marriage, and my life will always end in suffering. But I don't want the same suffering for my children. They need their mother around.

Yvette's reflections on her personal situation were pervaded by complaints about weakness. Apart from possibly reflecting a very real and physical experience, these complaints expressed her worries regarding her social status. Paradoxically, while excessive physical tolls had made her weak like an old mama, socially she had become like a child again as she had lost control over the assets that define proper womanhood: childbearing capacities and a productive field (recall that the Gbigbil word for weakness [*tekaa*] denotes not only old age, but also fragile childhood). Since her "old body" would prevent her from fulfilling the ethics of production and reproduction in the foreseeable future, her reentrance into childhood seemed almost irreversible—symbolized by the decay of her formerly productive field, the last tangible proof of her earlier respected womanhood. Whether comparing herself to an old mama or to a small child, what is clear is that Yvette considered her condition to be at odds with what was expected from her at this moment.

These same complaints, however, also served to defend her position. They formed a symbolic idiom with which she could allude to her virtuous womanhood and wifehood, and denounce the vicious attitude of Claude and his kin. After all, in line with the village's ethics of production and reproduction, she had depleted her force level for the sake of her husband and in-laws, while the latter, despite all her sacrifices, had not properly taken care of her. Rather than being the culprit in this whole story, she was the innocent wife who had endured the whims and woes of conjugal life.[14] This implicit counterattack was not without effect; as the above-mentioned reaction of Frédérique already showed, Yvette's rhetoric resonated well among some Gbigbil women. All witchcraft rumors aside, I also heard quite a number of women express their pity, sympathy, or admiration for Yvette.

In her attempts to reestablish herself as a respectable wife, the ethics of production—the agricultural and household tasks that she was now so eager to fulfill—came to overshadow those of reproduction. To justify her nonreproductive stay in her marriage, Yvette downplayed the virtue of childbearing. She also redefined it: sexuality and reproduction, once the cornerstone of marriage, were recast as *conditional*, rather than unconditional, conjugal duties. Not "blind conceiving," but rather consciously avoiding sex, using female-controlled contraceptive pills, and discontinuing childbirth had become moral acts. They turned her into a *responsible* wife and mother in an environment that had increasingly criticized her *irresponsible* sexual and reproductive behavior—especially since her last pregnancy.

Her wish to care for her living children and to leave them with an inheritance should be read as another claim to responsible motherhood. Drawing on the widely accepted "truth" that mothers offer their children the best love, care, and education, Yvette justified her motherhood *and* her stay in this marriage. The meaning of marriage became reformulated in the process: rather than the formal framework in which women are supposed to bear descendants for their husbands' patriliny, marriage was seen as the best environment for the creation of matrilateral and emotional ties between mothers and children. Focusing not on child*bearing* but on child *rearing*, and stressing her hard work in the fields as the only means to take care of her children, Yvette altered the ethics of production and reproduction in such a way that her current position and pathway into the future became meaningful for both herself and others.

Clearly, Yvette's reproductive interruptions implied a string of turning points in her reproductive life, accompanied by the constant redefinition of her position and projects. For others, similar experiences may involve less dramatic changes, or even be downplayed as nonevents. But all reproductive interruptions exacerbate tensions that inhere in women's status as rural women, wives, and mothers. Preventing the fulfillment of the ethics of production and reproduction, they threaten a respectful position and future in this rural setting. Women have various options to remedy such an ambiguous situation: they may get pregnant again and reduce conjugal conflicts, or go back to their families and find another marriage. If they do not have the physical and the social capital to explore these horizons, they may still redefine the nature and causation of the reproductive interruption (by strategically denominating what was lost and why), as well as its consequences for their position (by strategically altering the ethics of production and reproduction that lies at its basis), and, in this way, succeed in their quest for rural status.

Yet, as we will come to see, not everybody in Asung aspires to rural respect. The next chapter explores the dynamics of reproductive interruptions happening when women have abandoned the ethics of production and reproduction in favor of urban horizons.

Urban Horizons

4

Viviane, it's you who has done this to me
Viviane, it's you who has emptied my pockets
[. . .]
I have given my car; no, you didn't come
You have even taken my house; no, you didn't come
[. . .]
Every day she comes to say, "Give me the sum of money
That I will use during the week"
I give her my money, the next day she comes back again
"Give me again the sum that you gave me;
I owed money to a friend, she has demanded [it], I gave it back
Please, give again"
She cries for money; I get it out, I give [it]

—Song "Viviane," sung by the Cameroonian
artist Prince Aimé (my translation)

If men tell you they love you, they have already calculated something on you
If men tell you they love you, they have found something to profit from you
Men are like judges: you think he only treats your case,
    but he treated many other cases before
Men are like tailors: you think he only measures you,
    but he made many other clothes before

—Gbigbil song, sung to me by mama Rosie

THE VILLAGE IS ONE THING, the city another. Irrespective of whether this is actually the case, it is a strong conception that guides the daily life navigation of the Gbigbil people in Asung. It informs their day-to-day praxis as well as the potential futures that they imagine for themselves. For them it is clear: while a successful rural life can be attained through fulfilling the ethics of production and reproduction, a future in the city is associated with other pathways and projects. At some point in their lives, they may even try to explore these pathways and projects; while "searching their lives," they may switch their focus toward the urban terrain that they perceive to be so different from Asung's fields and the associated arena of activities and aspirations.

This chapter will highlight how the meanings and management of fertility change along the way. In the face of urban horizons such as schooling, employment, or profitable urban relationships (rather than fields, fire, and fertility), Gbigbil women may have different intentions regarding marriage and motherhood. The navigations of pregnancies and their interruptions vary accordingly. Reproductive navigation thus takes a different form here because the horizons and aspirations are different—not necessarily because the women or reproductive events are fundamentally dissimilar. Owing to the existence of both rural and urban imaginations in Asung, the story of Sophie, which will illustrate the importance of urban projects during certain reproductive conjunctures, is as likely to be found in the village as the stories of Yvette and the others mentioned before. Taken together, they provide insight into the different modes and patterns of navigation arising around Gbigbil women's critical reproductive conjunctures.

Sophie's Story

My first visit to a marabout. Together with my informant Sophie, I am sitting on the floor of a small room in the house of the female Islamic healer, who silently watches us while we wait for her son Abdullah to join us for translation. Unable to communicate with her, I wonder what she actually thinks about this unannounced visit of an unknown client and her white anthropologist friend. Though her face does not reveal any surprise or disapproval regarding my presence, I feel intensely self-conscious. When I received Sophie's invitation to accompany her here, it felt like a great opportunity to experience the secretive practices that so many informants had so often mentioned to me; now, however, I feel uncomfortably out of place. The awkward silence, and the train of reflexive thoughts it provokes in me, comes to an end when Abdullah enters the room. After he orders

Sophie to pass some coins to the marabout, the divinatory consultation starts. Immediately, the marabout starts posing questions in Fulfulde, translated by Abdullah into French:

Abdullah: Your husband, did he marry another girl?
Sophie: Hmm-mm [she smiles meaningfully at me]. You see?
Abdullah: Do you have any problems with your husband?
Sophie: Hmm-mm.
Abdullah: You are not with him, are you?
Sophie: Hmm-mm, I am not in his house.
Abdullah: How did that come to be? Why did you leave the house?
Sophie: Well, for the moment it is because I am ill. I came to my family
    because I am ill.
Abdullah: But your husband asked you to come back, isn't it? And you
    don't want to go back, do you?
Sophie: Hmm-mm. I am afraid.
Abdullah: Who gave you the medicines for your body?
Sophie: The medicines for my body? I went to the hospital and searched
    indigenously as well.
Abdullah: What do you want her to do?
Sophie: I would first of all like to *know*, since I am ill . . . Because when I
    am staying with my family, I am in a good state as you can see me now.
    But when I am there, together with my co-wife, I am regularly ill, it is
    not going well, there are problems; a lot of things.
Abdullah: She says there is a thing that they sent on you and that you have
    to treat.
Sophie: So . . . this thing, is this just on me or is it really in the house, the
    same house?
Abdullah: It is in the house. She says that you should not go back to your
    husband like this, without making some medicines.
Sophie [to me]: Erica, you see?

A few months before, Sophie had temporarily come to live with her mother next to my house in Asung. She was unwell and claimed to need some rest. Not ill enough to be bedridden but not healthy enough to go to the fields either, Sophie had ample opportunity to spend her time with me. Over many tea sessions in her mother's kitchen, Sophie shared the worries that, according to her, would make her lose even more weight if she did not talk about them. Gradually, I gained insight into what had preceded her illness episode.

Sophie had been born, some twenty-seven years before, as the third daughter of the fourth wife of her influential father, who worked as a *chef de poste agricole* in Asung.[1] One of her thirty-six siblings, a daughter of her mother's co-wife, had remained childless in her marriage and fostered Sophie when she was five years old. Next to her sister's lessons in and around the house, Sophie also had the chance to enjoy formal education in different cities; as the husband of her sister had a mobile job, Sophie was taken along to Bélabo and the capital of Yaoundé, where she did well in class. After finishing her primary education, her father, who had the financial means and the ambition to get all his daughters properly instructed, sent Sophie to secondary schools in the cities of Bélabo and Bertoua—an unusual but increasingly popular opportunity for girls at that time. Sophie loved especially her dactylographic courses, where she discovered her "talent" and came to imagine a future as a typist. But then her father became seriously ill. The money that had enabled Sophie to pursue her education was now invested in his hospital visits and operations. School was over for Sophie.

In this indecisive period, in which future prospects were destroyed and Sophie experienced her daily activities as being "without any goal or development," she became receptive to the temptations offered by boyfriends. Presented with their gifts and financial rewards, Sophie "started to like the taste of it." Not long afterward, at the age of seventeen, she conceived in a relationship with a married and jobless man who tried to "search his life" in the city:

> He just helped me out, bit by bit, until the moment he would "have" me. And then, it was over. For me, that pregnancy really came as an accident. I thought, "If my father will hear that I'm pregnant, what will happen?" And my friends would make fun of me. I was so ashamed. So I told my boyfriend that I would search for people who would give me remedies to abort the pregnancy. He said that if I would do that, I would die. In that way, he cursed me and that made me afraid. I was forced to keep the pregnancy.

Next to this fear, the lack of money and knowledge of abortifacients hampered the realization of Sophie's abortion wish. When her boyfriend eventually gave her money and told her to go to the hospital for a pregnancy termination, most of these constraints suddenly seemed to disappear. His offer turned out to be a pretext to get her to attend prenatal consultations, however; considering the advanced gestational stage, the doctor instantly refused an abortion and proposed a medical follow-up of Sophie's pregnancy instead—something her boyfriend had apparently anticipated. Even if this incident disappointed Sophie, it helped to appease the reaction of her parents. Although they did not like the news, what mattered most to them was that Sophie's boyfriend had assumed his (financial) responsibility and care for their daughter's pregnancy. This is not to say that they expected anything *more* from him, though. Instead, they strongly supported the explicit marriage refusal of Sophie, who wanted to "ensure her future" first. Especially Sophie's father, who had invested his financial means in his daughter's education, clearly envisaged another future for Sophie than this "down-and-out" guy (*va-nu-pieds*) could probably offer her. He insisted that even if there was a child, Sophie should still go to school or work without being burdened by mothering tasks or by entry into marriage.

These ambitions were quickly realized when, soon after the birth of her daughter, Sophie found a teaching job as a dactylographer. She went to live with her maternal grandmother in the city, who took care of her baby whenever Sophie went to school to teach. Sophie's motherhood did thus not interfere with her daily activities or projects for the future; to the contrary, it even played a decisive role in the relationship with the man who would eventually become her husband. Seeing the "proof" of her fertility, Alain became interested in Sophie. As he really longed for children at that moment—being the only child of his mother, and having no descendants since he had been together with several infertile women—he quickly started preparing the traditional gifts to her family as soon as Sophie carried his pregnancy.

However, the then eighteen-year-old Sophie considered herself too young to bear another child. Unlike a first child, a second child would make an educational future very unlikely, and given the enthusiasm of Alain and his parents, it would potentially tie her to a marriage. She tried hard to abort the pregnancy but failed. Afraid to die after three attempts to open her cervix, she eventually decided to keep the pregnancy. After all, if a marriage would ensue, it would offer her a privileged position: Alain had an official job as a teacher at a missionary school and could satisfy her needs with his financial capital, while she could satisfy his and his parents' need for children with her childbearing potential. These prospects eventually also made Sophie's parents agree with the situation. The birth of a daughter, the quick transfer of medokh meyal (the wine of birth), the resulting "friendship" between Sophie's father and father-in-law, and Alain's tactic to move Sophie into his house in the city soon afterward, finally concluded the marriage.

One month after she weaned her second daughter, Sophie became pregnant again. She was excited about it. "As I was a married woman now, it was good to bear a lot of children, even a hundred." However, she miscarried after two months. She related the incident to me as follows:

> My miscarriage was caused by the women's worm that often roams in the lower abdomen.[2] It started biting me when I was already pregnant for two months. When I wanted to urinate, I saw some spots of blood. Although my aunt gave me some barks [of a medicinal tree] to stop the bleeding, it did not help because the worm was alive. I should first kill it. It is the Mectizan medicines that have treated this for me.[3] I had gone to the hospital to ask if the Mectizan that we should take would only kill simple worms. They told me that it even kills the women's worm. I decided to try to take this, and it killed the worm. The same month I got pregnant again.
>
> My husband was angry when he heard that I miscarried. He thought it was me who had tried to abort this pregnancy. I told him, "No, of course I know the methods, but I could never do that. It is a worm." I also told this to his family members who asked me about the cause. And then they saw it themselves, because I got pregnant immediately after I took the Mectizan. That's what they wanted. In the end, they didn't consider it too much, since it was a pregnancy of two months that contains only water.

Her next pregnancy, bringing another daughter, was gladly received by Alain and his parents. They even started to talk about formalizing the union at the municipality in the near future. With the prospect of a marriage certificate, which would allow her to "profit even more from his wealth," Sophie was happy to conceive again in the hope of quickening this process. It was during this fifth pregnancy, however, that, as Sophie told me, "everything got spoiled." Alain's attitude toward Sophie and her children changed drastically; he was absent most of the time and disregarded his financial responsibilities.

It turned out that he was seeing another woman—who was married, had four children, and would even have a son with Alain. Although Sophie accused the woman of falsely claiming that Alain was the father of her son in order to win his attention, Sophie saw that these lies *did* have an effect on her husband. Alain even denied being the father of Sophie's pregnancy, while taking full responsibility for "that child outside that is not even his." Seeing no positive prospects whatsoever and thinking of the burden of her three daughters, Sophie tried to abort the pregnancy with natural remedies but failed again. As her female relatives and friends whispered that abortions were risky, that children "do not last," and that married women should give birth irrespective of the circumstances, Sophie decided to keep what she later called her "pregnancy of suffering."

The particular reason behind the change in Alain's attitude long remained unclear to me. Posing the question directly to Sophie only provoked heavy accusations toward her co-wife, who Sophie claimed was using charming powers in order to totally possess Alain. When I asked her about the role her in-laws had played in this affair—knowing that tensions in marriage often involve the husband's kin as well—she once again turned the attention to the evildoings of her co-wife: her in-laws strongly disagreed with the situation and reproached their son for having taken a second wife, but the charming power of this woman made their words ineffective. Sophie downplayed any potential frictions between herself and her husband or in-laws. She turned all attention to the tensions with her co-wife instead.

It was only when she participated in one of my focus group discussions that I gained a more nuanced understanding of the behavior of Alain and his parents. The discussion focused on the relationship between mothers-in-law and daughters-in-law, both competing for the attention of one man. To my surprise, Sophie cried out that she would advise everybody to marry a husband without a mother, because mothers are so greedy and men are obliged to give in to their wishes. She explained how her own mother-in-law, having only one son, wanted to compensate for her lack of children by fully exploiting Alain: not only did she claim part of his salary at the end of every month, but she also encouraged him to have mistresses who would offer her services and grandchildren. I was stunned to witness the ease with which Sophie publicly shared this information that had never appeared in our interviews. It shed a different light on my previous interactions with her; I started thinking more critically of what she had told me and what not, and how this reflected the actual issue at hand. Though I understood that Alain's extramarital relationship might indeed have been inspired by his mother's (or parents') search for descendants, his unwillingness to recognize Sophie's pregnancy remained surprising to me. If they were so desperate for children, he would have been more than willing to embrace the new pregnancy of his wife.

That there was even more to the situation I discovered after an unexpected incident. One morning, Sophie and I were waiting for one of the haphazardly passing cars to take us to an indigenous healer, while drinking tea inside. Seeing a car pass by at high speed, Sophie started loudly regretting that we were not outside at this moment, since the taxi driver was actually one of her recent lovers. Surprised, because she had never mentioned her extramarital affairs to me in our conversations, I asked her whether she had many such lovers. Unequivocally she answered, "Yes of course, since my husband was only floating outside, I decided to search "ma part" as well." It turned out that Alain had refused to acknowledge the pregnancy because he suspected her to have conceived with one of these lovers.

Though the relationship with Alain improved once Sophie's fourth daughter turned out to be "his picture" and paternity could no longer be denied, problems with her new co-wife increased after the latter moved into the house. Rather than "suffer inside," Sophie ran away several times, seeking refuge with her older sisters and mother in Asung. From this time onward, her mother becomes more visible in Sophie's narrative. Having been raised by her sister, Sophie did not seem to have had a particularly intimate bond with her biological mother during childhood. Things had changed, however, after the death of Sophie's father. Disputes over inheritance with the sons of her three co-wives had made Sophie's mother return to her own brothers on the other side of Asung. Here, her relationship with Sophie improved. Both women defended each other's interests now: Sophie, as a "sister's daughter" (mo kal), had the traditional position to demand certain privileges for her mother in her maternal family, while her mother acted as an important marriage broker and safe haven for her daughter.

Nevertheless, despite her help, Sophie's mother insisted on Sophie's eventual return to the marriage. She had various reasons for doing so: she was subjected to the demands of her brothers, who could eventually contest the prolonged stay of their mo kal in the compound; she herself felt burdened by her regularly returning daughter and grandchildren; and, most of all, she would be more likely to receive some bride-price payments (especially the "money for the mother") if Sophie endured in the marriage. Thus foreseeing an unpreventable return to her husband, Sophie started to secretly take contraceptive injections in order to prevent another pregnancy with him. Like many other Gbigbil women in this area, she preferred the three-monthly Depo Provera injections over the daily ingestion of contraceptive pills as risks of forgetting and of discovery by the partner would be considerably smaller. Yet, at some point she herself did forget to attend a follow-up consultation and became pregnant right away. It was within this context of conjugal turmoil that Sophie experienced another miscarriage:

> It started with pain in my back, around the kidneys. It got really warm. I went outside, because I thought that I wanted to urinate. When I squatted, a ball of blood fell down. I stayed for at least thirty minutes in the WC because the blood was flowing. Then, I stood up, went to the house, and changed my clothes. My husband neglected me, as always. I suffered a lot afterward and bled a lot as well. So my husband told me, "Take this money and go to the hospital for some injections." There, they said I suffer from typhoid. But even now that I am under treatment for this typhoid, my belly is very warm inside. Why doesn't it go away if I take the proper medicines? And look, when I am here in the village, far from my husband and that woman, the situation tends to ameliorate. But when I get back in the city, in my house, problems worsen again. I will never enter that house again as long as that woman resides there. I will not bear children anymore.

Although this second miscarriage occurred at a similar phase of pregnancy as the first one, Sophie's experiences were clearly dissimilar. Asked to compare the two events, she reflected:

> There is really a difference. The first time, we found out [about the cause], we treated it, and it cured me. I never encountered the problem again. But this time, even until now, I still feel the pain. And it remains very warm inside. I don't know. I would like to finish the typhoid treatment in the hospital. And then, I will go and see ahead. Because she [her co-wife] practices day and night, and she succeeds in it. And I only practice during the day.[4] I searched [for indigenous medicaments] here in the village, but

that doesn't work well. It tends to help a bit and then it releases again. So what I want is to go to a marabout. I will hear everything that she [her co-wife] is doing, and I will be treated.

Indeed, our visit to that female Islamic healer proved to be a turning point in Sophie's illness episode. She confirmed that Sophie's co-wife had charmed her husband and practiced witchcraft to destroy Sophie's fertility and conjugal future. She gave Sophie remedies for restoring her health and childbearing capacity, for making the co-wife's harmful remedies affect the co-wife herself, and for making her husband listen to her again. Sophie's search for help had become a contest for power: deprived of financial and social security within the conjugal sphere, she felt compelled to make use of the marabout's offer to "combat the evil with evil"—the only promising horizon that would enable her to regain her powerful position as a first wife within her urban marriage.

One year later, I found Sophie living together with her daughters in a small wooden apartment in Bélabo, paid for by Alain. She happily related the effects the healer's interventions had had: her physical ailments had disappeared, her co-wife had remained childless ever since, and her husband seemed willing to listen to her wishes again. He had even proposed to try to have another baby together. Sophie took this as a hopeful sign; she claimed that a pregnancy would enable her to regain her position as a first wife in Alain's house and fantasized about the subsequent departure of her co-wife.[5] Once things would be "settled" like this, she would finally be able to continue with her dactylography training and find a real job. Half jokingly she exclaimed, "I need a typewriter to get started, and where will I find the money if I'm not even close to my husband?"

New horizons and hopes asked for new reproductive politics, and a rethinking of former ones. Sophie reassured me that, from now on, she would cling to her new project: "I decided that I won't go into another marriage. I am here, and I wait for him. I exerted my politics by always keeping my children with me. Unless I die, I know he will always come back, because I have his children. Men just want children, and so they become children themselves: it is easy for a woman to play with a man in that way. I know that I will conceive, and I know that I will be fine in the end." Even if Sophie's final depiction of her complex experiences as just "a play" may seem simplistic and only part of the story, many urban marriages in this area are in a way indeed a "bet"—with different aspirations and stakes involved.[6] The nature of such "bets" can be understood only if we know what attracts Gbigbil women like Sophie to urban areas in the first place, and what the "rules of the game" are once they enter this zone. The following will therefore describe Gbigbil imaginations of, and encounters with, urban life and its potentialities—of which marriage and reproduction are just a few.

Urban Aspirations and Pathways

Gbigbil people are in many ways confronted with town life. Some, like Sophie, move beyond the rural realm from a young age onward. Parental liaisons or flexible fostering practices make them accustomed to a mobile lifestyle, in which they regularly stay in urban households and encounter educational, biomedical, juridical, and religious institutions in the surrounding neighborhoods. Others may decide to "search their lives" in the city only after having spent considerable time in the village. With Bélabo and Bertoua within reachable distance in both directions of the paved road that traverses the village (see Figure 1), and with Gbigbil acquaintances and bigger markets present in those two cities, they might, at some point, seriously consider following those who have preceded them. Whether from the beginning or only later in life, many Gbigbil people thus alternate their stay in Asung with periods spent in urban realms.[7] Their specific reasons for doing so are multiple. Yet, such moves are almost always inspired by the idea that urban life offers more attractive possibilities and future prospects than those encountered in the village.

As much as rural life is pervaded by the ethics of production and reproduction, urban life is considered its antithesis. Rather than to prioritize "work in the fields and births of many children," life in cities is thought to center on other activities that offer alternative future scenarios. My informants claim that its driving force is not subsistence but rather the accumulation of money. The pathway to respectability is not the exposure—and thereby, depletion—of physical force (ngul) but rather the exposure of financial capital and of social links with those who possess money. According to many Gbigbil women, a shift to this alternative frame of honor would ensure the preservation of force, youth, and beauty and would also give them more rest, more time, and more options with regard to productive and reproductive activities than could ever be attained in the village.[8] Even if ideas of an easy and honorable life in the city may not correspond to actual urban realities, such views and expectations *do* underlie people's decisions to leave the village and "search their lives" elsewhere.[9]

In this search, several pathways are believed to enhance the realization of urban ambitions. The first and most frequently mentioned route into city life is the educational one.[10] Ever since schooling became widely accessible for both boys and girls during the economically flourishing decades of the 1970s and early 1980s (Johnson-Hanks 2006, 2007), it has broadened the scope of ambitions and possible futures beyond the village level for men and women alike. With education perceived as a way to attain formal employment and modern honor, many Gbigbil parents, like Sophie's father, have come to consider the instruction of at least some of their children a worthwhile investment for an uncertain future.[11] Especially those children who show a particular seriousness or aptness during their first years of life are encouraged to develop their inborn talents and characteristics in school, and thus become a "real person" (*faŋ mod*) through self-realization.[12] This pro-educational stance is widespread in southern Cameroon and follows logically from the "wealth in knowledge" paradigm long existent in the region. Individual talents and characteristics were already an important source of power and respect in the acephalous groups that were scattered through the forest in precolonial times; on the basis of outstanding personal qualities and inventive activities, men could attract many followers and wives—and thus, gather "wealth in people" (Guyer 1996; Johnson-Hanks 2006; Laburthe-Tolra 1981).[13] Schooling enhances this process of becoming a "real person" in the current era, for men and women alike.[14] It offers new pathways to respectability and inspires aspirations to other forms of wealth and respect than those related to the village ethics of production and reproduction.

Second, it is through the job market that money, and thereby urban respectability, can be accumulated. The employment that is envisaged here is ideally formal and acquired through a certain level of education. In the current atmosphere of economic decline, however, a salaried job is an increasingly rare form of capital. Ever since 1994, the year in which the Cameroonian currency devaluated, civil servant salaries have drastically decreased (with cuts of up to 80 percent), and unemployment rates have been on the rise. Those who succeed in being formally employed are therefore likely to be surrounded and respected by the many others who did not; it offers them not only financial, but also symbolic and social capital. Even those who did *not* succeed in getting a formal job—people with a lower educational level, or those who are well educated but hampered by current high unemployment rates—might still be enviable from the villagers' point of view. They can become successful through inventive income-generating practices on the Cameroonian informal markets, which are dynamically related to state institutions (Geschiere and Konings 1993; Goheen 1993; Guyer 1996; van Santen 1993). Gbigbil women who have less experience with schooling than with work in the fields and in the kitchen may aim for exactly such a career. They become involved in small-scale trade, prepare dishes to sell at urban roadsides, or try to compete with urban traders by buying products in surrounding villages and reselling them in town markets.

Third, urban honor can be achieved through prestigious liaisons such as sexual relationships, marital alliances, kinship connections, or clientism with urban elites. For many Gbigbil women, the preferred pathway into an urban life is based on relationships with rich men who are established in the area. Through the money of these men, women may attain the luxurious and respected lifestyles they are aiming for; through the connections these established men open up to them, they may access formal jobs or other opportunities. The following will delve into the dynamics of these relationships and explore the underlying ideas and ideals of partnership and parenthood. What role do marriage and fertility play on the pathway to urban respectability?

The "Big Fish" Bet

Marital habits have long been in flux in the East Province of Cameroon. Chapter 1 indicated that marriage norms and expectations have probably always diverged from actual conjugal practices in the region; Chapter 3 exemplified how this discrepancy can work out in the village. Marital relationships acquire different meanings again in the face of urban horizons and alternative forms of honor. Where schooling, jobs, and money are present and explicitly aimed for, marriage ceases to be the only means to attain respectability. It seems to become relevant only *later* in life. Especially from the mid-1980s onward, there has been a visible trend of rising marriage ages for both men and women in urban areas all over Cameroon (Calvès 1999, 2000; Garenne 2004; Johnson-Hanks 2007). In 2011, urban women did not marry before they were twenty years old, while men waited until the age of twenty-seven; thus, they married three years later than their rural counterparts (DHS 2011). Consequently, premarital sexual relationships, which might or might not culminate in what is finally agreed to be a marriage, have proliferated in these zones.[15] Such relationships often attain different intensities, serve different interests, and acquire different meanings for Gbigbil women and men who pursue urban projects.

The most common and volatile sexual relationship is called a "simple friendship" (*amitié simple*). Such a "friendship" is constituted by a gendered exchange of food, sex, and money: men give money for food and other gifts, women cook for and sleep with men. Yet, the two "friends" do not live together. The relationship persists as long as some kind of reciprocity is maintained between the partners; clear future visions or further commitments are mostly absent. Women mostly stress the attention, gifts, and support these friendships might offer them. "We just want wealth," my informant Dianne once told her husband Baudouin when he complained to me that many women these days maintain multiple *amitiés* simultaneously. Indeed, if financial support is what is aimed for, the best strategy for women is to engage in "simple friendships" with more than one man. As these men may have several other girlfriends or wives, who all "demand their parts," they will face economic shortages now and then, or at least claim to do so. Not only "free" girls (*ngon si*) but also married women who feel financially unsatisfied with their husbands engage in extramarital "friendships" for this reason—provided that they veil their escapades in secrecy.

While such pre- or extramarital amitiés are common in both rural and urban areas, they acquire particular meanings for unmarried women who aim for a future in the city. These women often explicitly attempt to be involved with the most respected and well-to-do men in urban environments— preferably older men with formal employment. Such partners are called "big fish" (*gros poissons*); they are seen as "a good catch that could fill your stomach."[16] My friend Laura once explained, "Big fish are people like the prefect, the mayor, a commandant, or taxi drivers. We engage with them for the honor to live with somebody who earns money. It is not necessarily a marriage with them that we want." Instead, what they want is to attain an urban lifestyle through the material and symbolic advantages such friendships offer them. In this, they are often encouraged by their relatives. With the eventual transfer of a bride-price far from secured in the current era of economic and conjugal instability, family members try to profit from—if not some parts of the bride-price—the gifts and connections these "big fish" may offer their daughter and themselves.

Although explicitly sought after by women and their families, relationships with "big fish" are often surrounded by ambivalence as well. Owing to their wealth and status, these men are solicited by many women (and their families) alike and have to distribute their attention and money over multiple partners. Long-term relationships with "big fish" are therefore considered unfeasible; most lovers rather seek instantaneous advantages. As Laura noted, intense engagements are also not necessarily what women aim for; a hypothetical entrance into marriage is often conceived as a possible obstruction to other nonmarital ambitions. Consequently, as much as they are seen as a source of temporary pride and respect by women who wish to embed themselves in urban circles, these relationships are often considered by others—especially elders in the village—to be appalling examples of women "selling their bodies." Even relationships with "va-nu-pieds" (down-and-out guys), as Sophie called the father of her first child, which are all too clearly based on material interests or otherwise violate the reciprocal "rules of the game," might be labeled as despicable instances of *escroquerie* (exploitation) or *bordellerie* (prostitution).

This vision is also widely disseminated in the Cameroonian media. In 2012, a news article in the daily *Cameroon Tribune* warned that the phenomenon of prostitution is not only restricted to girls "from the street," but increasingly concerns youngsters, students, and even married wives who search for financial advantages from men.[17] Another article from 2014 mentions the problem of prostitution directly in relation to the high number of "free unions" and states that these should be combated by the Ministry of Women's Empowerment and the Family.[18] Women's financial exploitation of men is a prominent theme in Cameroonian music, too. In the song mentioned in the epigraph to this chapter, Prince Aimé (Beloved Prince) describes how he spent all his money on gifts for his demanding girlfriend Viviane, but was left alone and humiliated when he fell short of money. Online reactions to the clip on YouTube show a general acknowledgment by Cameroonian men and women of the depicted situation and reveal some moral ambiguities around the image of women's use of strategic sex:[19]

We women, we are very strong! We pretend to love whereas to the contrary, it is only the money that we love. Let's change our behavior.

What you are saying is very true!!!!!!!!!! People please beware of all the Vivianes.

Today everybody is Viviane in a way, even men. Let's pray every day that this spirit of escroquerie disappears, because it's better to take the money of a man that you love.

Cameroonian girls are Cameruinean, so what? Is it only us? Let us be!

Everywhere in the world women are the same. In fact, it is the nature of a human being. Too bad for the unlucky ones. Just use your brains and not your emotions.

While the first two reactions acknowledge but implicitly condemn Viviane's attitude, the latter two naturalize and celebrate it. As seen above, both extremes were uttered by Gbigbil people as well. The middle comment is more nuanced; it indicates that this behavior applies to both men and women, and to both relationships based on escroquerie and those characterized by love. It is exactly this nuanced remark that sheds light on the ambiguities of relations with "big fish," for, as much as the unconditional exchanges may constitute a factor of instability, they could serve as a basis for a "deep friendship" (*amitié profonde*) or "serious engagement" (*fiançailles*). The exchange of sex, food, and money is part of every intimate relationship in eastern Cameroon, whatever its duration and outcome. It is a cornerstone of relationships that are intended to be serious and long lasting as well. Male attention in the form of money and gifts serves, as it has long done, as an indicator of his potential as a future spouse; it is considered a proof of his love, responsibility, and serious intentions. Women's sexual relationships with "big fish" are thus ambiguous: while they can be instrumental for the achievement of other urban goals like schooling, employment, or pecuniary honor, their stabilization can at the same time become a goal for those who aspire to an urban marriage with a promising husband.

The sexual behavior of Cameroonian men shows similar ambiguities. Like their female counterparts, urban men have several reasons to postpone their marital engagements and keep relationships informal. Multiple, volatile sexual encounters offer them the possibility to "search a life" before getting married and having children; they may lead to financial benefits (especially from older, well-to-do women); they provide status among peers and family members, who generally value the display of masculinity and potency;[20] or they exist simply because men have limited capabilities to fulfill formal marriage obligations. This is not to say that these men do not value marriage in itself. While engaging in "multipartenariat," they are prone to search for the "best girlfriend," who might sooner or later become a spouse.[21] Apart from behavioral characteristics, women's educational level is hereby often explicitly taken into account. A Gbigbil student in Yaoundé explained his deliberations after he had interrupted our conversation when a young girl walked by. With a low voice, he had asked her whether she could tell her older sister that he wanted to meet her that night. When I inquired whether that sister could be considered his girlfriend, he said:

> Many girls here are *zam zam*: they go from one guy to the other and are not really serious. I don't like that. I want a serious girl and an educated one, like this one. I hope she will become my best girlfriend. But for now, I have several girlfriends. As a man you cannot stick to one girlfriend only. Maybe you say that she's your everything and that you only go for her. After some time, you might find out that she is not how you initially hoped she would be. She can display certain characteristics that you hadn't expected, or she seems not well educated. Briefly, you can't imagine a marriage with her. And then you have no alternatives. So it is better to have different girlfriends at the same time. And women do the same, you know.

Sexual relationships are generally fraught with mutual mistrust. While this might be true everywhere in Cameroon, it becomes exacerbated in urban settings, where alternative horizons create more independence between partners. The presence of alternative projects and the strong competition on a flexible marriage market where men and women aim for the most profitable partners, as well as a general lack of bride-price payments once engagements become more serious, all imbue urban "partner plays" with ambiguity.

This does, however, not do away with the *ultimate* goal of marriage in life, nor does it alter long-standing expectations of gendered reciprocity between potential marriage partners (and their families). To the contrary, the "commoditization of sex" before marriage and the value women attach to men's financial generosity should be placed not only in the current conjuncture of economic crisis—as transactionalist interpretations tend to place it[22]—but also in a historical context where "the social structure of marriage exchanges centered on bridewealth, in which a man's commitment to a relationship is measured in the frequency and extravagance of his gifts" (Johnson-Hanks

2007: 651). Even if long-standing gendered reciprocities may have become reconfigured into new *forms* of partnerships in urban zones, marriage as an ultimate *framework* for respectability remains intact. It is just no longer necessarily the only aspiration and is therefore part of a larger frame of projects. And so is fertility, as we will see.

"The Vagina Doesn't Talk": Flexible Motherhood and False Fatherhood

Charlotte: It is very simple to mislead men.

Dorine: Women in particular can easily mislead men, since women are wiser than men.

Charlotte: A man only knows that he has a wife. But he doesn't know how his wife often conceives a pregnancy.

Nadine: You only tell him you are already pregnant.

Charlotte: He will ask you when it has entered. It is up to you to tell him the day and the date that you did something together. And he will have to believe it.

Dorine: Haha, a woman? A woman is very strong!

Nadine: Criminal!

Angélique: First devil!

Dorine: Because there are things that a woman does and a man can never know. You pretend that you walk together, but . . .

Charlotte: If God will succeed to put me in a marriage, I will be with my husband. But when another man flirts with me and my heart also wants to go there, I will run very fast as soon as my husband is at a minor distance. And nobody will know what I have done.

Nadine: The vagina doesn't talk. And yet, it has already worked!

Although the above excerpt forms part of a focus group discussion on women's general forces and tactics, it is not surprising that the particular youngsters speaking here had all been in relationships with "big fish." It is especially in informal sexual liaisons with urban men that women's manipulation in affairs of love, sex, and reproduction is warranted. As these ambiguous relationships can dissolve as easily as they can lead to more formal engagements, pregnancies often have a major impact on the direction taken in the partner play. Depending on the circumstances and the aspirations at hand, they can do both—that is, either immediately disrupt a relationship, or stabilize it into a "deeper friendship" or even marriage. As fertility is not always explicitly aimed for, nor does it necessarily lead to subsequent engagement, pregnancies, even more than these sexual relationships themselves, constitute a "bet." The meanings and implications of conception for such relationships are subject to constant negotiation between the two partners and their families; once a pregnancy "enters," previous pathways may be rethought, new projects considered, and shifting situations manipulated.

For many women with urban aspirations, conception is perceived to stand in the way of the realization of their ambitions. The often-heard expression "c'est fini pour toi" verbalizes the idea that a pregnancy, just like a marriage, might prevent the fulfillment of one's projects and foreclose the horizons that had appeared on the pathway toward city life. Although pregnant youngsters in Cameroon are legally allowed to continue schooling after a maternity leave,[23] in practice many school-going women fear losing their educational opportunities—or subsequent employment chances, for that matter—once they are confronted with a pregnancy. Their worry seems justified by the reportedly high pregnancy-related dropout rates in secondary schools in Cameroon (Eloundou-Enyegue 2004; Eloundou-Enyegue et al. 2004; Lloyd and Mensch 2008). It is further reinforced by public advertisements against "untimely pregnancies" (*grossesses précoces*) that the Cameroonian media disseminate. One poster shows how, of two school girls called Clarisse and Angeline, the former ends up poorly after she conceives with a temporary lover, whereas the latter, who finishes school while abstaining from sex, faces a bright future as a good-looking, motorbike-riding (and thus probably employed) woman (see Figure 3).

It is the fear of ending up like Clarisse and missing the chances of Angeline that underlies the stories of my school-going informants relating (failed or successful) abortion attempts. These stories are omnipresent; abortion rates among school-going women in southern Cameroon are relatively high (Calvès 2002; Johnson-Hanks 2002a). This is not to say, however, that the link between school enrollment and fertility desires and outcomes is straightforward.[24] The entrance of a pregnancy does not automatically imply an entrance into motherhood or wifehood for Gbigbil women. Sophie's story showed how young women can send their children to their father's household or relinquish parental rights to other relatives to circumvent motherhood or wifehood and continue education after birth.

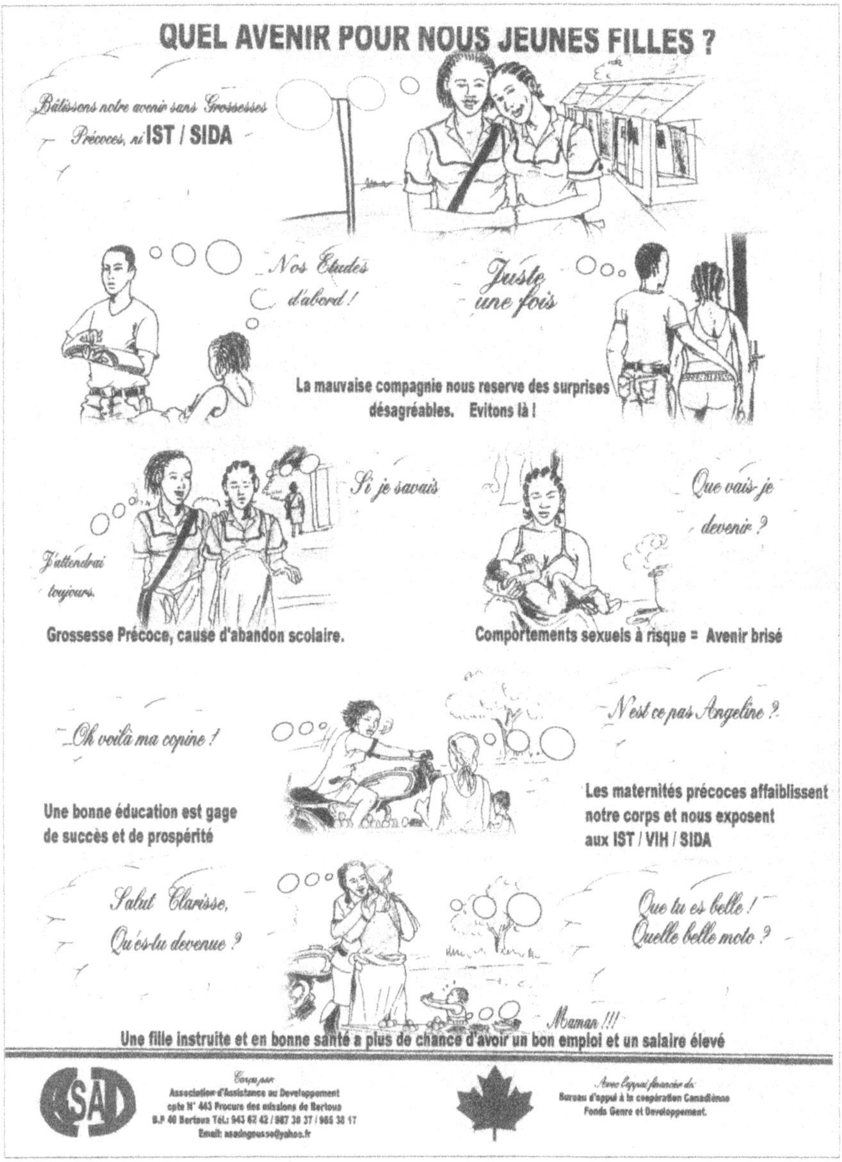

Figure 3. Poster warning against premature pregnancies. The headlines on the poster say: "Which future for us young girls?"; "Bad company reserves for us unpleasant surprises. Let's avoid them!"; "Untimely pregnancy, cause of school abandonment"; "Risky sexual behavior = broken future"; "A good education is a guarantee of success and prosperity"; "Premature maternities weaken our body and expose us to STD/HIV/AIDS"; "An educated and healthy girl has a better chance to have a good job and an elevated salary."

With sufficient social capital and support—from a partner or the family, or both—a pregnancy does not necessarily interfere with urban projects, even if it might initially be perceived to.

For others, a pregnancy forms exactly a means to realize urban ambitions since it may ensure financial support from and a symbolic link to a respected man in the city. When a relationship with a "big fish" seems profitable to a woman, a pregnancy might be a worthy attempt to "stick" this partner to her. One strategy is to conceive with him; another is to allot a pregnancy to him even if he is not the biological father. A woman who succeeds in convincing her rich partner of his fatherhood and gets him to openly acknowledge it expects herself to be more or less reassured of care, financial support, and increased contact during pregnancy and the first years of her child's life. In the current absence of bride-price payments (which used to establish a husband's paternal rights over all the children his wife would bear), a man can ensure his de facto right over his descendants by acknowledging his paternity and providing financially for mother and child (see also Chapter 1). Mere impregnation is not sufficient; fatherhood should be socially achieved. Women "play" with their partners—especially those expressing a wish for children—accordingly. The experience of Charlotte, a pretty Gbigbil woman who worked in a city bar and was tellingly nicknamed "the hot one," resonates with the stories of many others:

> When it was still a pregnancy of one or two months, I told my sisters, "Don't tell anybody. I myself will know to whom I will give my child. Then, I won't suffer anymore like I suffer now. If the guy really wants a child, he will look after me and the child." There were two of them in Bertoua. One was married and the other was not. So I asked both of them for the layette—both the father of my child and the other whom I had also told that he had impregnated me. Both of them have come, hey! We first saw a car arrive with soap, fish, and meat. And then the second father of my child came with a car full of food as well. Sacks of rice, boxes of soap, food, fish, meat, everything! Just to come and see the child. He thought it was his child and we didn't want to deny it. So we said, "Here is your child. Do you see how he resembles you?" He looked at the child and said, "This is my blood." Haha, I thought, "Ah, if only you knew." Oh, I have played with men! But my people have drunk, my people have eaten.

Charlotte did not envisage marriage per se; she contented herself (and her family) with the material benefits as well as the symbolic liaisons that this allotment of her pregnancy could offer her. She capitalized on the wish for offspring that several promising lovers had apparently expressed, without necessarily expecting further formal engagements.

Other women *do* try to enforce marriage once they recognize a certain willingness in a man to engage—even if he is not the biological father of the child she is carrying. In these cases, what is aspired to is the honor of being married in general (for, as stated, marriage remains an *ultimate* framework of respectability, also in cities) or of living with an urban "big fish" in particular. In order to attain these marital goals, women may tactically deploy an age-old norm that links childbearing to a marital framework; they posit marriage as the unpreventable outcome of a pregnancy conceived in an urban affair. Although this norm is mostly not adhered to in practice, women do resort to it in an attempt to alleviate the uncertainty of their indeterminate relationships. This is what Sophie suspected her co-wife had done: by claiming her child to be Alain's, she had managed to find her way into marriage.

It is also what my informant Joséphine decided to do, after overcoming her initial fear that the pregnancy she conceived with a well-to-do, married lover would "spoil her future" in Bertoua. Once this lover had openly declared that he "did not want to flee from the pregnancy" and assured his accountability in front of her family members, Joséphine decided to "profit from the child that links us already." She said she would insist that the father of her future child would pay her education and help her find a job. Even if that meant she would have to marry him, she would do so. "What can I do? We already have a child." Although marriage was thus presented as the unpreventable outcome of this reproductive conjuncture, it might in fact have been the most promising horizon at hand for Joséphine. A marriage had become a desirable new project because it could safeguard her urban aspirations; her pregnancy was used as a first step in this direction.

Some others go even further: they take their ambition of an honorable urban marriage as the starting point and strategically disclose their pregnancies accordingly—in the hope that at least somebody in the city would take fatherhood as an incentive for more formal marriage arrangements. Nadine's story shows how her pregnancy was turned into a possible pathway to an urban future even before concrete horizons in that direction had appeared:

Nadine had borne six children with four men and had lost one girl and all of her three boys. Her two remaining daughters were living with her ex-husband. The death of her last son had triggered a situation in which she was left with no children to care for, no stable relationship with the boy's father, Didier (considered her informal "husband"), and no clear future perspectives. When she was offered a job as a servant in Douala, Cameroon's economic capital, Nadine gladly accepted and left the village behind to "search her life" in the big city. Finding only hard working conditions and many poor lovers unwilling to assume a responsible relationship, however, she decided to return to her natal village nine months later. Here she detected not only that Didier had had relationships with two other women, but also that she herself had missed her period. She realized she had conceived with a married man she used to go out with in Douala.

After an initial wish for an abortion of what would become a "bastard child," Nadine decided to keep the pregnancy. Her pregnant state would enable her to undergo treatment for the affliction (*iwò*) that she suspected had caused her previous children's deaths.[25] Further, this pregnancy would help her find a marriage somewhere in a city; as gossip about her marital instability abounded in the village, Nadine wanted to restore her honor through marrying a respected man elsewhere. This would also prevent her child from being the "bastard child" she feared it would otherwise become.

The question was thus to whom to "give" her pregnancy. Three men entered the stage: next to the biological father from Douala and her socially recognized husband in the village, she thought of the driver of the car she traveled in on her way back from Douala. A man without a wife and with a formal job in the provincial capital, this driver quickly turned into one of Nadine's lovers worthy of imagining a shared future with—more than the two other men at this moment. The man in Douala, Nadine contemplated, would never believe in her being pregnant; instead, he would suspect her of inventing the story to receive money. A formal engagement with this married man was highly unlikely. Didier, on the other hand, had proven to be promiscuous and was moreover based in the village—a place that she seriously considered leaving now that it was associated with deception, child death, hard work, and gossip. She therefore concluded, "If the chauffeur wants to continue, I will tell him he should take me, including my pregnancy. But not now, because we just started and he will not believe this pregnancy is his. I have to wait a bit first, then reveal my pregnancy, and see what he decides."

Starting her treatment itinerary while still contemplating about a possible father, Nadine was told by an indigenous healer that, to heal her affliction effectively, she needed the cooperation of the father of the pregnancy—which was assumed to be Didier. Owing to his physical proximity and her desire to be treated, Nadine switched focus and told Didier that the pregnancy she carried was his. Didier initially agreed to cooperate but retreated when he later heard gossip about her having conceived the pregnancy in Douala. With no other men in the direct neighborhood to run to, and with the burden of shame and family curses caused by her capricious marital behavior, Nadine decided for an abortion. After some failed abortion attempts, though, Didier begged her to keep the pregnancy, despite his ambivalence regarding his paternity. A future marriage with him was again envisaged and negotiated: Didier proposed to fully engage once a blood test on the newborn baby would confirm his paternity; Nadine demanded his faithfulness and their relocation to the city.

However, when Didier traced several of Nadine's lovers on her mobile phone, his uncertainty about his paternity was exacerbated, and he broke all contact again. This, together with the subsequent curses Nadine received from several family members, strengthened Nadine's wish to leave the village forever. When she coincidentally received a phone call from the taxi driver, she immediately told him she carried his pregnancy. The man was overwhelmed and asked her for time to reflect. In this undecided period I asked Nadine about her hopes for the future, whereupon she answered: "The ball is still turning. My chance will fall wherever it falls. If it is with Didier, I will return there. But he knows my conditions: I decided not to work in the fields anymore and to go to the city instead. Even if he doesn't agree, I will leave. And if I succeed at the other side [i.e., with the driver], I will block him [i.e., Didier] for sure. It's very simple: if a man gives you a pregnancy, and you see that he's not well situated, but you see that another one is better off, you can balance them. So I balance the two and will see where it will end."

Over a period of only a few weeks, several opportunities and obstructions presented themselves to Nadine. She constantly adapted her ambitions with regard to fertility and marriage accordingly—without, however, losing sight of the bigger urban aspirations that she aimed to realize through this pregnancy.

Though some pregnancies may seem to be strategically anticipated, many women do not make a priori decisions or calculations about marriage and childbearing. Most of the stories of my informants show how things just happen without anticipation, how their own wishes or future visions are often unclear and inconsistent, or how their pregnancy-related projects are shaped only after conception by the decisions of their family members and partners. Relatives influence the negotiations around sexuality and reproduction considerably. Even if they are located some distance away in the village, they often actively interfere in the reproductive affairs of their promising daughters, for whom urban pathways had been anticipated. In line with their own needs and aspirations, they reject premarital pregnancies, or they encourage them; depending on their own situation, they focus on the financial responsibilities of the father, or they align a child to their own family. Sophie's story shows that the same holds for parents-in-law, who may influence the marital choices and fertility wishes of their sons who have become "big fish," and thereby also those of their girlfriends and (potential) wives. Women's reproductive navigation should therefore always be considered in the light of the social web of relations established *before* and *during* the reproductive conjuncture at hand.

This navigation is also influenced by the behavior and intentions of male partners. Like their female counterparts, Gbigbil men may have multiple aspirations at the same time—contrary to the Gbigbil song in the epigraph and patrilineal idioms that proclaim a persistent male desire for offspring. A pregnancy may be considered a burden by those who still want to "search their lives," who lack financial means to raise the future child properly (since "everything needs to be paid for in the city"), who have money but prefer to spend it on other things, or who do not feel like engaging with the woman who claims to be pregnant. Reluctance to acknowledge paternity may also derive from their recognition of women's maneuvers with regard to motherhood and wifehood. After all, it is only the woman who knows for sure whose pregnancy she carries, and to whom she wants to "give" it. It is this worry that bothered all three appointed fathers in Nadine's story.

Confronted with a pregnancy of which they are not certain to be the father, or to want to be the father, men have several options: abandoning the pregnant woman, acknowledging the relationship, acknowledging the pregnancy, or acknowledging both. With no formalities established, no financial obligations yet fulfilled, and often even no relational stability, men are relatively free to decide what to do when they are appointed as future fathers. While this is the case for men with rural and urban aspirations alike, a study by Calvès (2000: 452) shows that this decision seems most related to the desirability of conception and the characteristics of the union.[26] Paternity is more likely to become contested by men with urban aspirations or in informal urban relationships—even if contestation also occurs in the village or, as Alain's sudden misrecognition of Sophie's pregnancy illustrates, after a considerable amount of time has been spent together and childbearing has become a common project.

Men who explicitly aim to find (or keep) a suitable marriage partner and/or her children acknowledge that there is little that they can do to prevent "false fatherhood." Some try to calculate the menstrual cycle of their wives or girlfriends as accurately as possible. Others, like Nadine's "husband" Didier, threaten to conduct a blood test on the newborn baby—which they almost never do in practice. Still others, such as Sophie's husband, who rejoiced in the fact that his last daughter turned out to be "his picture," rely on the "force of blood," which will either show common physical traits between father and child or direct the latter to its biological genitor even years after birth. Finally, those who are desperate for children resign themselves to the fact that women have a final say in these affairs; since "the vagina doesn't talk," it is only the talk of the woman that counts. Baudouin, who returned to the village after several relationships with urban women who appeared to be infertile, explains:

> Most men are just happy to follow the words of the woman: "He is the one who gave me this pregnancy." You are just proud to hear that this child belongs to you. Even if there are ten men . . . girls of these days "balance" men. The one has a bit more means, the other is too poor. Even if it is the poor one who made her pregnant, she will say that it's the other. And since we [men] are lonely, we are thirsty for children. Even if we have ten [children], we always want even one more. So when they come to tell you that "You have made me pregnant," it always brings joy. You know that you have another child. Even if, in reality, it is not yours.

This pattern of "selective recognition and support" (Calvès 2000: 446), in which various options and degrees of paternal acknowledgment are possible, differs substantively from former times in which bride-price payments automatically ensured paternal rights over the children born in a union—even those conceived with another man outside of marriage. Once men had initiated their bride-price exchanges, all the children their wives would bear would by default belong to their lineage. "Bastard" children, even if ranking lower socially, would still have a place of belonging in society.

Nowadays, with the decrease of bride-price payments, and with several law reforms that disconnect legal partnership and paternity from monetary matrimonial exchanges,[27] fatherhood needs to be explicitly acknowledged in marital unions that are not legally established—that is, the majority of current Cameroonian conjugal relationships.[28] The conclusion for the children born in such unions is that "whether the parents have actually concluded a marriage is considerably less important than whether a man is willing to acknowledge fatherhood and to claim the social and economic responsibilities of that role," as Bledsoe and Cohen (1993: 80) have observed. Paternal recognition is crucial in establishing the economic status, social identity, and access to wealth and inheritance of children born in unstable unions. However, urban men who have other projects than parenthood in mind may be reluctant to recognize a child. Without any recognition, these children are more likely to be raised by their maternal grandparents or by their mothers, who, despite their urban ambitions, often lack formal employment or other sources of regular income. While the dependence of these children on their maternal family members is in some cases wished for, in many other cases it is not. Nadine's insistence on finding a possible father out of fear of bearing another "bastard child" proves that, even if *bâtards* are commonplace these days, the fate of these children is often as unsure as the (urban) relationships in which they were conceived.

Negotiations around the unborn fetus are thus plentiful. They define the fate of many uncertain urban relationships and pathways. Reproductive interruptions have a similar decisive force. The next section will situate "wasted wombs" in a context in which partnerships and parenthood are only part of a much larger frame of urban projects.

Fetal Fights

Just like the conception of a pregnancy, the interruption of a pregnancy reveals the stakes and ambitions that are inherent to urban relationships. In uncertain unions, pregnancy interruptions are always imagined *possibilities*. Apart from those instances in which women actually resort to abortion (discussed in the next chapter), they may *threaten* to interrupt their pregnancies for multiple reasons. First, it can be a way of putting more pressure on a man to engage. If he was initially not eager to accept paternity, the prospect of the removal of the unborn fetus may persuade him to do so—either for the sake of the child or for the sake of the relationship with the woman. Thus, invocations of a possible abortion become a means to "test" a partner's intentions. Yves, a male informant who was in the process of becoming a "big fish" for many women, encountered such a situation. During one of our conversations, he received a phone call from a girlfriend, who told him that she had aborted the pregnancy she claimed to be his. After a long story about how the two of them had maintained an informal sexual relationship in urban hotels, he related:

> At a certain point she called me to say that she was pregnant. From me. And if I wouldn't take her in the house, she would abort it. I told her, "Do not abort, because that is risky and you could die." But I also told her that she couldn't come and live with me. I have a wife and four children, and that's enough for me. I told her so. Because maybe it was just her way of binding me to her. Maybe she had conceived with another man and told me that it was me, because she wanted to marry me. Well, and now she just called to say that she has evacuated the pregnancy. She asked me [rhetorically] whether she could have really kept it, in this situation. Well, that's fine with me. Thank God that she succeeded without any problems.

Second, a woman's invocation of abortion may be a tactic to receive money from a rich partner who is clearly unwilling to engage, or with whom she herself is reluctant to intensify the relationship. Whether or not this money is actually used for an abortion is contingent on subsequent situations or reflections. The next chapter will show how my informant Laura, for instance, started prenatal consultations with the money she received. Men, in turn, also find ways to tactically negotiate the demands for abortion money by their pregnant partners. We have seen how Sophie's first boyfriend gave this money only in such an advanced stage of the pregnancy that doctors would surely refuse the abortion and start prenatal consultations instead. Both men and women can thus use the hypothetical option of pregnancy interruption to pursue their projects within (and beyond) the ambiguous partner play. In this, they flexibly deploy existing embryological notions, which on the one hand consider a beginning pregnancy to contain only "water water," but on the other hand acknowledge the gradual development of a human being (see Chapter 2). Shifting interpretations of what a pregnancy actually is inform negotiations of why it should be kept or "evacuated," and negotiations of its implications for one's relationship and future personal projects.

When such interruptions become an actuality, then, these questions become even more relevant as they determine the degree of eventfulness of the reproductive happening. In line with their particular projects, women and those surrounding them can either downplay the interruption as a noneventful "late" or "disturbed" period, or turn it into an event with clear causes and consequences. The first option is often deployed when women fear that public knowledge of their pregnancy interruption would interrupt their wider urban ambitions—for example, schooling that is financially supported by one's parents, or a relationship with a "big fish" who seems to long for offspring. Especially if they have a mobile lifestyle and maintain volatile relationships that do not imply a constant copresence of partner, co-wives, in-laws, or relatives, women have more possibilities to hide and dismiss their blood loss than if they are permanently settled in the village.

Sometimes fertility interruptions cannot or should not pass unnoticed. Once a pregnancy interruption is conceptualized as such, it becomes enmeshed in negotiations and explorations of possible causes. The etiological repertoire is vast; people might invariably invoke the will of God, heavy work, abrupt body movements, numerous diseases (both "indigenous" and "biomedical"), malediction, the administration of indigenous remedies (by themselves or by malevolent others such as jealous co-wives or female competitors), or (their own or others') witchcraft (see further van der Sijpt 2007; van der Sijpt and Notermans 2010).[29] These different naturalistic and personalistic etiological categories imply various degrees of culpability and possibilities of accusation; they therefore constitute a flexible idiom that can be differently employed at different moments. Depending on the social situations and personal aspirations, women whose pregnancy has been interrupted can turn the attention either to something negligible ("work" or "the women's worm"), to an abstract agent ("God" or "the witches"), or to specific people with whom social relations have been distorted ("my jealous co-wife" or "my mother who cursed me").

Such tactical etiological explanations are even more warranted since "wasted wombs" raise implicit questions of one's *own* intentionality. When asked what could possibly interrupt a pregnancy, most Gbigbil people imme-diately noted that most "wasted wombs" are in fact provoked by women them-selves. Such induced abortions are often presented as miscarriages; as a result, spontaneous interruptions are often suspected to be provoked. The unclear intentionality behind most "wasted wombs" blurs a strict divide between spon-taneous and induced loss. To portray oneself as a passive sufferer of external causes of loss may be a woman's tactic to reduce suspicions and to divert atten-tion from her own potential intentions underlying pregnancy interruptions.

While such etiological manipulations happen everywhere, they become of specific relevance in relationships with urbanites, in which pregnancies are from the outset surrounded by more ambiguity and mistrust. Since fer-tility is often not the primary aim of either partner, since multiple alter-native aspirations and loyalties are clearly present, and since abortion methods are generally better known and accessed in town, the possibility that a "wasted womb" might in fact be induced by the woman herself is, if not explicitly acknowledged, always implicitly suspected. This is not to say that women necessarily abort their pregnancies more frequently when they have urban aspirations and lifestyles than when they do not. Rather, it demonstrates the degree of distrust characterizing interactions between partners who find themselves in a zone of multiple horizons and who are uncertain about the other's reproductive goals. Reproductive interruptions thus confirm *and* exacerbate the distrustful ambiguity that surrounds fer-tility matters in such relationships.

This heightened ambiguity is not always disadvantageous. It can offer both partners room to negotiate their stakes in the social situation at hand. The indeterminacy of the causes and consequences of "wasted wombs" allows for many possible outcomes of the reproductive conjuncture. It offers people space to bring their pathways in line with their aspirations—urban, marital, reproductive, or other. However, not everybody can exploit this ambiguity fully; certain forms of capital and other conjunctural circumstances define which options are available and perceived to be feasible or attractive. The last section of this chapter will illustrate this point, by analyzing the different dynamics informing Sophie's reproductive navigation.

Negotiating Hopes and Horizons

While the previous sections have depicted possible marital and reproduc-tive options for Gbigbil women with urban aspirations, particular forms of fertility management can be fully comprehended only when situated within the specific reproductive conjunctures in which they occur. Contrary to a common depiction of urban women—or women with urban aspirations, for that matter—as individuals having required a certain independence in (reproductive) knowledge and decision-making, I agree with Bledsoe, Casterline, et al. (1999: 14) that also for them "a certain fertility dynamic has been set up well before the women themselves take any reproductive decisions." Which fertility dynamic had been set up for Sophie, then, and how can we make sense of her navigation of the different reproductive conjunctures in her life?

As Sophie was born as the third child of the fourth—and youngest—wife of her father, many siblings (from different mothers) had preceded her. Most of them had already borne children as well. Motherhood was therefore not presented as a priority for Sophie; since the quartier was already full of descendants and her relatively wealthy father envisaged alternative futures for his children, she was neither expected to bear children for her own lineage, nor obliged to quickly do so for a family-in-law. Sophie's mobile lifestyle, exposure to urban influences, and attendance of different schools during the years in which she was fostered by her sister further enhanced an image of future womanhood inspired by ambitions beyond those of rural production and reproduction. Motherhood and wifehood were not only potentially postponed, but also made part of a larger repertoire of projects. This amalgam of aspirations offered Sophie room to negotiate different ambitions and interpretations of fertility and marriage at different points in her life.

Her two premarital pregnancies were associated with very different interpretations of motherhood. Initially, the pregnancy conceived in the informal "friendship" with the father of her first child was anxiously equated to motherhood and marriage with a va-nu-pieds—considered final obstructions to a still hoped for future educational path. The failure of Sophie's abortion attempt and the influence of her parents, however, led to a reconceptualization of the implications of this pregnancy. Stressing the temporary character of pregnancy and nursing, they rather minimized the consequences of childbirth for other future projects. In the face of alternative horizons they concluded that now was not the time to become a (socially recognized and enacted) mother or wife: neither the present circumstances nor future images suited that. Pregnancy was one thing, motherhood another.

A different view of motherhood appeared when Sophie conceived with her husband-to-be Alain. Despite her initial abortion considerations, the wish for children of both Alain and his family made her reconsider the value of this pregnancy in the absence of any other hopeful horizons for the future. After all, with his salaried job as a teacher, Alain was a good "fish" to catch. The pregnancy suddenly turned into a means to bind an influential man to Sophie and enable her to still attain a form of urban respectability—a project that had become increasingly endangered by the sickness and financial shortcomings of her father. The marriage that resulted did not erase her previous ambitions related to educational and personal development; rather, these were put in a different time frame. Instead of postponing motherhood for the sake of education, this unanticipated marital situation made Sophie postpone her educational ambitions for the sake of motherhood. Her priority was now to give some children to this "big fish" who seemed desperate for offspring, in the hope that it would offer her marital respect and financial security (especially through a marriage certificate), as well as the possibility to continue schooling afterward.

Sophie's aspirations changed when conjugal conditions worsened and promises of urban respectability (as the only wife of a "big fish") and financial comfort (through a legal marriage) vanished. Anger about a sudden unfaithfulness and the neglect of expected duties by her husband pushed Sophie to take "revenge" by also depriving Alain of what he expected from her: children. Her repeated stance that "I don't refuse to give children, but I won't give them in such a situation" transformed a married woman's duty to bear children for her husband into a *conditional* one. The mere *context* of marriage was not enough to make Sophie unconditionally adhere to the childbearing norm; the *content* of the relationship also mattered to her. The possibility to make such a firm fertility-related resolution seems based on several forms of capital that she possessed. After all, she had borne some healthy children for which she knew Alain was longing, she had found alternative lovers who could financially maintain her, she had a safe haven in the village where her mother and sisters would allow her to come and "take rest," and she had an educational foundation that would, even in the absence of a marriage, allow her to search for employment and thus an alternative source of urban honor.

Yet, over time, most of these alternatives seemed less advantageous than anticipated. Acknowledging that support from her own kin had become limited since her widowed mother resided with her own family, that relationships with outside lovers were not able to give her the long-term prospects that she could find "inside" a marriage, and that she could draw on her dactylographic knowledge only if she owned a typewriter, Sophie turned her fertility into a project again: as her co-wife had remained childless, conception would revive Alain's (and his parents') interest in her and assure her reentrance into marriage and her restoration of urban respectability. Such sudden changes in perspective show the importance and complexity of conceptions about the "right" timing of childbearing, motherhood, and wifehood, and how these are negotiable and changing—contingent on previous pathways, present circumstances, and projects for the future. This not only applies to the *entry* into motherhood and wifehood but extends *beyond* initial childbearing and marriage. Since it is women's aspirations that inform the appropriateness and appreciation of their pregnancies, it is not surprising that women with multiple but uncertain urban aspirations—which might switch to rural projects again at any point in time—shift their notions of the right timing for motherhood and wifehood throughout their life course.

Shifting fertility aspirations also underlie Sophie's management of her two "wasted wombs." These happened in two completely different social situations. In the first instance, Sophie had been the center of attention of her promising husband and in-laws, who seemed able to offer her a comfortable urban lifestyle. Given their strong desire for offspring and the earlier conflict between Sophie and Alain's childbearing intentions, the pregnancy interruption raised suspicions of induced abortion. To appease the distrust that now characterized the relationship with this promising "big fish," it was in Sophie's interest to externalize the cause of her misfortune by exploiting a "neutral" etiological discourse regarding the "women's worm." After showing her "goodwill" and "innocence" by killing the worm and conceiving again, the incident was soon disregarded.

During the second pregnancy interruption, the situation was almost the reverse: Alain had turned his attention to another wife and no longer cared about Sophie's childbearing capacities; he neglected Sophie and her family financially; Sophie's ambitions of a future formal marriage had been destroyed by the arrival of the co-wife; and becoming pregnant was something that she initially had not hoped for. This "wasted womb" revealed Sophie's marital insecurities and her reproductive (in)competence in the current conjugal competition. Not surprisingly, Sophie externalized the cause of the interruption and depicted herself as a sufferer again, but with totally different connotations: simplistic, naturalistic explanations—like the "typhoid" diagnosis she received in the hospital—were no longer adequate but were replaced by personalistic accounts of the co-wife's witchcraft practices. These accusations and Sophie's active search for remedial counterattacks show how the event became a trigger for Sophie to publicly denounce the insecure marital situation and to reassert her ambitions. What was at stake now was the preservation of the union with, and loyalty of, a "big fish"—the only feasible horizon toward a restoration of urban honor.

Together with a shifting etiology, notions of embryology shifted in such a way that this second incident became much more consequential. This time, what was lost in early pregnancy was no longer negligibly described as "only water" but was considered a potential human being and even Sophie's childbearing capacity in general. Yet, her repeated utterance of "I will not bear any children anymore" remained highly ambiguous; it could indicate the undesirable consequence of affliction as well as a conscious decision to stop childbearing. Maintaining this ambiguity around the intentionality of her interruption allowed Sophie to strategically shift positions and power relations: sometimes she lamented her lasting dependence on others in marital and reproductive domains, while at other times she implied her "fertility halt" to be a deliberate way of punishing her husband. Contrary to Yvette, who, as described in the previous chapter, tried to downplay all ambiguity connected to her fertility interruptions, Sophie turned this ambiguity into a resource. Indirect allusions to induced abortion strengthened her demand for marital responsibility from her husband and in-laws. She was able to utter them because of the presence of supportive family members as well as her record of successful childbearing and conjugal dedication. Unlike Yvette's story, Sophie's case has shown how reproduction and interruptions can turn into opportunities to denounce certain circumstances and assure individual aspirations—especially when women possess different forms of capital such as a respected background in the village, education, employment, childbearing capacities, or living children.

Sophie's pregnancies and their interruptions were pervaded by changing and sometimes even contradicting feelings, rationalizations, and ambitions—even if her wider project of living in the city remained intact. The presence of alternatives and of different forms of social support and capital offered Sophie freedom for these interpretational shifts. Pregnancies turned from unwanted to wanted or vice versa; contraception was introduced and stopped; interruptions were sources of grief or relief. Contrary to what family planning campaigns and posters like the one shown in Figure 3 (targeting educated young women) presume, fertility desires are never stable but—especially in unstable partnerships and during unstable pathways—change flexibly in accordance with one's hopes and horizons, and the negotiations thereof during reproductive conjunctures. In the face of multiple, quickly changing horizons, Sophie's reproductive decisions were "bets" on an uncertain pathway to urban respectability.

The stories of Sophie and all the other Gbigbil women that have appeared so far have illustrated the different projects that may be pursued at different moments in life, and the ways in which these projects are at stake when "wasted wombs" possibly derail previous (rural or urban) pathways. They have shown the new horizons that may appear during reproductive conjunctures on these different pathways, and I have analyzed *why* women might prefer to explore one or the other. The next chapter will look at reproductive navigation with a different question in mind: it sets out to describe *how* women make, negotiate, and justify their navigational choices within the particular webs of social relationships in which they are embedded. It will show that, irrespective of their particular trajectories and choices, women often have a common way of portraying their projects to those that surround them—with paradoxical effects.

Discourses of Decision-Making

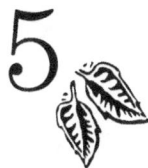

There exists a contradiction between the theory that women have no voice and the fact that some of them "speak."

—Philippe Laburthe-Tolra, *Mínlaaba: Les seigneurs de la fôret*
(1981: 900, my translation)

REPRODUCTIVE NAVIGATION IS FULL of decision-making. Those decisions can be implicit or explicit. They can be covert or overt. And they can be part of improvisation or the result of conscious deliberation. No matter their particularities, they underlie the uncertain process of plotting and actualizing reproductive trajectories that reproductive navigation is. This chapter aims to shed light on some general discursive devices that women deploy while navigating reproductive conjunctures—irrespective of which direction they want their pathways to take, which hopeful horizons they wish to explore, or which personal projects they aim to pursue. It explores not *why* they make particular choices, but *how* they go about framing, asserting, and justifying these reproductive decisions within the social worlds of which they are part. As such an exploration, this chapter aims to unravel broader patterns of interaction between individual women and their social surroundings, and the ways in which these interactions help women navigate their reproductive conjunctures.

The shared idioms of distress, destiny, and decision-making that are central to this chapter shed light on the common pool of navigational narratives deployed by Gbigbil women with different reproductive experiences and aspirations.[1] But they also challenge common Western assumptions *about* this navigation. First of all, they question the application of a suffering-agency divide to different forms of interrupted fertility; generally, spontaneous loss

139

and infertility are associated with suffering, and induced abortions with agency. Second, they challenge prevailing discourses of modernization and empowerment that portray rural women as merely powerless and their urban counterparts—or those with urban ambitions, for that matter—as powerful.

The stories of a village mama experiencing secondary infertility and of a young, educated, and urban-centered woman attempting to abort several pregnancies serve as a starting point for this chapter, because they would, according to the above assumptions, represent clear instances of suffering and agency respectively. However, I will throw a different light on this supposition by illustrating how both women use images of power and powerlessness in a similar way—despite their different pathways, reproductive experiences, and projects. Further, as the two cases could be considered two extremes on a "reproductive continuum," they form a starting point to generate more general insights about reproductive navigation and the ways in which (inter) personal characteristics affect its outcome—something that will be discussed more elaborately in the conclusion of this book.

Hanging Underwear: Mama Rosie's Story

Mama Rosie is one of the most prominent mamas in Asung; it is difficult for both outsiders and insiders to ignore this woman with her heavy body and loud voice, who lives right in the center of the village. Her slow pace caused by painful and rheumatic knees stands in marked contrast with her quick uptake of, and eager participation in, multiple activities in the village. As the *présidente* of the women's association Seying ining (We search our lives) she is the one to inform and organize women around crucial events in Asung and its surroundings;[2] as an *agent de santé* she is a regular visitor of all households in order to measure and promote mother and child health;[3] as an in-married wife in Asung she is renowned for her performances during village palavers and funeral ceremonies;[4] and as my "adoptive mother" she offered me delicious meals and secret knowledge on a daily basis. My regular presence in her household allowed me to closely witness her personality, problems, and actions; our frequent conversations introduced me to the circumstances, worries, and decisions that had shaped the previous fifty-two years of her life.

Unlike her complaints regarding her current marital situation, mama Rosie's stories about the polygamous family she was born into, in a Maka village some forty kilometers from Asung, are pervaded by good memories. As the third child of the second of her father's three wives, she grew up in an extended family in which "you could not know who was the mother of which child, because no distinctions were made." Things changed, however, after her father died, when mama Rosie was eight years old. Her mother left the marriage and remarried soon afterward. Only the first wife—taken through levirate (widow inheritance) by her brother-in-law—stayed in the compound and took care of the thirteen children of her deceased husband. The resulting "suffering," as mama Rosie called it, induced this *maratre* to write a letter to her former co-wife to convince her to come back and take care of her own five children, among whom mama Rosie was the only girl. Life became good again for mama Rosie; with not only her mother(s) but also many older brothers around, she was well taken care of and sent to primary school and a Catholic household school.[5]

It was only at the age of seventeen that mama Rosie started to menstruate. Freed from her worries about the absence of a normal menstrual cycle, she now initiated a sexual relationship with a primary school teacher who had been pursuing her for some time. After she had "started to like the taste of it," as mama Rosie smilingly told me, she neglected her schooling and engaged with Etienne, the son of the village catechist. The true "love relationship" that developed between them made him initiate bride-price payments, whereupon she moved into his house. "I thought that this was the man whom God had given to me," mama Rosie admitted with some regret in her voice. However, Etienne's mother, who argued that it took too long for mama Rosie to conceive with her son, opposed the relationship and proposed an albino girl who had already given birth elsewhere. This proposal was met with resistance; Etienne fled the village by joining the army, while mama Rosie's family members came to take their daughter back home. Nevertheless, the two lovers continued to write and occasionally meet in secret.

During Etienne's absences, mama Rosie engaged in sexual relationships with two teachers at the same time, Bernard and David. She conceived with Bernard at the age of twenty-one and rejoiced in the fact that, four years after the onset of menstruation, she had finally become pregnant. Bernard, however, left the village for a position elsewhere soon after mama Rosie had discovered her missed period. Etienne also put an end to their secret relationship as soon as he detected the pregnancy, and he married mama Rosie's maternal aunt instead—even though his mother, seeing the pregnancy that she had long hoped for, claimed that he must be the father and should take mama Rosie back into marriage. Although mama Rosie explicitly declined this marriage proposal as her aunt already resided in his house, she did not contest the claim of Etienne's paternity. "What could I say? Since we are in the same village, they could do wrong to my child if I would have said that it was not his. It is only God who knew to whom the child belonged." Since the biological father had disappeared and Etienne was engaged in a new marriage, mama Rosie decided to also tell her other lover David that he was the father. "I had to cling to somebody who could endure me with my pregnancy." David was willing to engage and came with the layette after the birth of mama Rosie's son. His marriage proposal was nonetheless again declined by mama Rosie; "I didn't want to marry anymore, because my first husband had deceived me and the father of my child had deceived me as well."

Thus disappointed by men, mama Rosie started to focus on her work in the fields, petty trade, the care of her son, and her job as a housekeeper at the Catholic missionary station in Abong Mbang, some fifty kilometers away. "I provided for my own soap and didn't think of men anymore. What can men offer me more than what I offer myself with my own hands?" Nevertheless, three years later, papa Gerie, who regularly visited a relative in mama Rosie's village, convinced her to come into marriage in Asung. As a descendant of the rather influential Bibakung family, he was known to and recommended by mama Rosie's aunt, who had gone into marriage in Asung herself as well. Having one son and one daughter from a deceased wife, as well as two daughters with a wife "who showed small weaknesses in her habits," papa Gerie was searching for a new wife "who would be able to cook for me," as he recalled to me later. As he agreed to take care of her son and to transfer gifts to her family, mama Rosie finally decided to "go and see."

Her arrival was met by the enormous resistance of her co-wife mama Cathérine. Heavily supported by her mother-in-law, who originated from the same village and who had arranged her marriage with papa Gerie, mama Cathérine accused mama Rosie of using indigenous remedies to take away her husband's love and her own position as a first wife. Many public judgments ensued in which papa Gerie's influential brother Albert—functioning as deputy mayor at the municipality of Bélabo—tried to ease the conflicts between mama Rosie on the one hand, and mama Cathérine and his mother on the other. Both in these *assises* and in her conversations with me, mama Rosie portrayed herself as a benevolent daughter-in-law who passively suffered the whims of her co-wife and in-laws. Her fertility problems reinforced this image of suffering:

> I entered menopause at the age of twenty-nine, after four years of
> marriage. Before this menopause, I didn't feel any pain in my belly.
> Nothing. My menstruation just stopped. You should have seen my
> breasts! The milk was even flowing. One would say that I was pregnant.
> Mama Cathérine feared that if I would bear a child for her husband,
> she would lose her place. But the pregnancy didn't come out. Only
> the breasts. People mocked me, and my co-wife's family accused me of
> inventing a pregnancy. Others suspected me of having aborted. I went
> to the hospital in Bertoua. They injected things to induce my period. It
> didn't come. I even went for an ultrasound in Ngaoundéré [capital of
> the Adamaoua Province]. They told me that I don't have a problem, that
> I should normally menstruate. They advised me to visit the traditional
> healers, because this was not at their level. And the traditional healers
> said that it is mama Cathérine who has blocked my menstruation.
> That she has taken my underwear stained with menstruation blood
> and attached it somewhere through witchcraft, so that I can't conceive
> anymore. Really, I suffered a lot. But what could I do? I was only lucky
> because [my in-laws] knew that I had given birth before. So I was not
> sterile. I arrived here when my child was three years old. So people
> couldn't really talk about me.

Whether in-laws and villagers *did* talk negatively about mama Rosie's childlessness or not at that time remains unclear; but surely mama Cathérine was put in a bad light by the accusations of different marabouts and mama Rosie. According to the latter, the accounts of hanging underwear were even confirmed by villagers who had seen her co-wife visit local healers to "attach remedies"—something mama Cathérine eventually publicly confessed.[6] Mama Rosie thereupon stopped searching for treatments, since nothing had ever worked and her husband had reassured her that he could not refuse her because of her childlessness:

> I decided to leave everything up to God. My life is in His hands. If
> it's God who made it stop, I will endure. If it's my co-wife, God will
> judge her. Because God himself has wanted people to be fertile and to

multiply, so it should not be blocked by others. But since I had love for my husband and he took care of me . . . If I made remedies to kill her, these remedies would also have killed a lot of innocent people. I have been baptized, and I cannot kill. I have love for God. And I have a heart of pardon.

This heart of pardon was questioned, however, by many outsiders who were prone to recall the serious problems mama Rosie caused when papa Gerie took a third wife a few years later. Many stories recount how mama Rosie wanted to kill this co-wife with a machete and was sent back to her family—after years of marriage that had in fact *always* been pervaded by struggles and fights. Mama Rosie, who had initially hidden this incident from me, admitted the case when I asked her about it; but rather than elaborating on the exact cause of the separation, she focused on the reunion with her husband one year later. She interpreted his demand for reconciliation as a sign of her own worth and indispensability within her family-in-law and the wider village. Encouraged by her relatives and this idea of personal significance, she had firmly decided to "regain my place in marriage and never leave again."

Indeed, her immediate accusation of harassment by mama Cathérine and the new co-wife helped her to reestablish herself. It led to the departure of the third wife, as well as papa Gerie's refusal to have sexual intercourse with mama Cathérine—who had just given birth to her fifth child—for the rest of his life. The situation improved for mama Rosie; after some time, papa Gerie even married her officially. Who exactly initiated the request for a formal marriage and whether mama Cathérine also obtained a marriage certificate remains contested. According to mama Rosie, it was papa Gerie who had wanted to consolidate their union and, in order to prevent problems, had proposed a formal marriage to his first wife as well.[7] However, in contrast to mama Rosie's own relatives, who had considered the acte de mariage a source of security for their childless daughter, the family of mama Cathérine had refused to sign the certificate as long as the bride-price for their fertile daughter was unpaid—thus leaving mama Rosie "the only wife in the household with a marriage certificate."

Although the lack of an acte for mama Rosie's co-wife was denied by papa Gerie and mama Cathérine herself—both claiming that a marriage certificate *did* exist—what is clear is that, over time, mama Rosie's position in the village and family-in-law solidified, while mama Cathérine's condition gradually degraded into a situation that was openly pitied by many villagers. Looking dirty and angry, walking barefoot, dressed in old rags, never going to the fields, rarely preparing food, and always carrying around her mentally retarded granddaughter who was allegedly "spoiled" by witches, she was said to "have no voice anymore" and believed by some to have been mystically "destroyed" by mama Rosie. Both her predicaments and my close connection to her rival mama Rosie made it almost impossible for me to approach mama Cathérine for a casual talk. Numerous attempts to investigate her points of view generally ended up in futile conversations full of uncomfortable silences; it was the price to pay for my allegiance to my "adoptive mother." Yet, one day, I succeeded in initiating a more open discussion about her current marriage. Although she did not directly invoke suspicions of her co-wife's witchcraft herself, mama Cathérine somewhat guardedly acknowledged her own downfall to me when she said:

> I don't like it. I had everything. Before, my husband wasn't poor like he
> is now. When a second wife comes to spoil the marriage, it is never good.
> But there are already children, and I wanted children. Rather than leave, I
> stay. People would say I'm not even here. I only watch everything with my
> eyes, I take care of my children and wait for my grandchildren. You need
> patience in polygamy. If another woman enters and you see that she has
> a high heart [*un coeur haut*], you should only lower [*abaisser*] your own
> heart. You should stay calm while the other speaks loudly. It doesn't make
> sense to insert your own mouth as well.

Others admitted more openly that my "adoptive mother" was considered a great witch in the village—for many reasons. First of all, mama Rosie's lack of children and absence of a normal menstrual cycle were considered suspect; "maybe it is because her witchcraft eats all her blood inside," some informants speculated. Second, mama Rosie's "power to speak" while she had rendered her co-wife mute must have been a result of her occult powers. Third, papa Gerie's preference for his infertile second wife over his fertile first wife must have been caused by the former's malevolent use of remedies. And finally, even my daily interactions with her were interpreted by some as a sign of the mystical powers she had exercised over me. Hearing this made me realize that my close connection to mama Rosie might have made not only mama Cathérine, but also other villagers uncomfortable talking to me. Thus, I became more cautious when mentioning or accompanying her in the village and at times even distanced myself from her a little.

Mama Rosie never contested this powerful image, or the fact that her co-wife was worse off than herself. She just explained it differently:

> I always knew that God would punish my co-wife. And there she is now, punished by God. It is difficult for her to even have five francs or one piece of soap. For more than five years, she hasn't been working in the fields. And I, I help myself. Even if I'm ill, I go to the fields. It is me who feeds her children every day. And these children come to me as well; they fetch water, they search for wood, they do everything for me. I leave everything up to God. But I know I also have this power that my family-in-law gave me. The women who firstly arrived as wives in this family have a lot of power because they are the eldest. With their own power they can tell me, "I was the first to arrive here, and I give you my power to govern." That's what they did. They appointed me as the president of the women's association. They gave me a power that makes all people listen to me when I speak. And there is also my brother-in-law Albert. When I arrived here, I gave him a lot of respect. I always gave him the first products of my field [*tjang*].[8] When I did this, he told me, "Even if I die, you will always govern my quartier." That's why, even if there were problems with my husband, Albert always wanted me to stay. Because he had already appointed me as the governor of his quartier. It followed from my good behavior. Albert said that I am the one who helps to raise the children. I am hospitable to the visitors. I have good habits. I prepare a lot of food. The whole family eats. So I am a wife of the family. And it is the work that you do in front of the people and your husband that makes a marriage and that makes you a woman. Even if you don't bear children.

Thus confirmed but also contested, mama Rosie's powerful position had always been surrounded by ambiguity. The sudden death in 2007 of her thirty-year-old son, who had lived with his biological father ever since Bernard had come to claim his child, exacerbated this insecurity. "Formerly, I knew that if somebody insulted me, my child was alive and would come and defend me at a certain point. But now, even if somebody wants to hit me, who will respond for me in the place of my son?" That there was much more to it than only physical defense became clear to me during a chat with my informant Laura, her father, and her blind uncle. While discussing general problems of polygyny, these neighbors and classificatory brothers of papa Gerie started to denounce mama Rosie's behavior as they had witnessed and interpreted it over time:

Father: Their marriage certificate was even signed in secrecy after mama Rosie had asked for it herself. Imagine! And afterward, papa Gerie said that, since his own children do not [officially] belong to him, mama Rosie's son will be his heir.

Laura: And now the child is dead.

Uncle: A deception created by God. God has seen that if He would leave things to happen, it would end very badly.

Laura: God doesn't forget anybody. You do your things and think you have won, but you don't know what will happen to you later.

Uncle: To the contrary, you will lose.

Laura: She has lost. She doesn't even have any grandchildren. Mama Cathérine's children will stay with the wealth of their father. Mama Rosie wanted to take this, but she didn't succeed.

Uncle: Rosie doesn't even have any right to speak if papa Gerie dies.

Laura: She really doesn't. Government is government; family is family. The family will decide. And the government cannot do anything at this level. They don't know anything; they can only hold a pen and write. But we know everything here in the village. Who will accept her?

Father: A woman who leaves her own village to come and dominate another village . . .

Uncle: It's the force of remedies! She is a bad demon—a real Satan.

Laura: And that's how many people who say they love God are. Those who are often in the church are the greatest witches. We're afraid of her. And therefore, she's all alone. Eke.

Like many other villagers, these neighbors pointed to mama Rosie's increased insecurity with regard to her inheritance rights. Now that mama Cathérine had one son and mama Rosie had none, the latter, even with a marriage certificate that she claimed her co-wife did not have, would possibly encounter problems upon her husband's death. The recent deaths of papa

Gerie's siblings and eldest son made the question of inheritance even more pressing and radically altered the prospects and positions of both co-wives. To be sure, mama Rosie was both literally and symbolically one of the biggest mamas in the village now; surrounded by many foster children, namesakes, and people demanding her advice during my evening meals in her hangar, she would proudly state that she was "the mother of everybody" or would be called "my wife of *ambiance*" by papa Gerie. However, whether this ambiance will continue after his death is something "only God knows."

In many ways, mama Rosie's story reveals dynamics and contingencies that we have seen before—with her particular pathways and projects directing her particular reproductive and marital decisions. But the way in which she *talks about* and *justifies* these decisions is more than only particular; it also appears in the narratives of many other Gbigbil women—even those with more room for reproductive decision-making or with alternative (urban) ambitions. All of them invoke suffering and agency in similar ways; mama Rosie's story is, contrary to what one would maybe expect, not more about suffering than theirs is about agency. There seems to be a common narrative framework that is used by women with different social backgrounds, different reproductive experiences, and different ambitions alike.

To shed light on this narrative repertoire I continue to present the story of somebody who can be considered mama Rosie's opposite: Laura. As an educated young woman aborting pregnancies while building up a life in the city, her life course and conditions are clearly dissimilar from those encountered by mama Rosie. Yet, the framing of her reproductive experiences is not. Her story will therefore allow for the exploration of common languages of distress and decision-making that pervade and direct women's navigations of a variety of reproductive conjunctures.

Falling Mangoes and Falling Fetuses: Laura's Story

It is a chilly morning in August. After an icy trip on a motorcycle taxi, which brought us to the city center, I descend from the vehicle together with my informant Laura, who wears a blue dress with a pink flower print and carries a pink handbag. We quickly enter the labyrinth of unpaved paths in the neighborhood where we have an appointment with a mutual acquaintance. Laura reciprocates greetings from others but leaves questions about our direction unanswered. I ask her whether she feels nervous; her answer is negative.

Upon arrival at our destination, we find that the man in question has unexpectedly left his house—which from the outside looks so similar to all the other houses in this slum area. While waiting for him, we watch—together with some children, patients, and neighbors—a soap opera on TV. Laura, like the others, reacts animatedly to the plot of a certain Anita trying to spoil the marriage of her lover Deniz. She seems to feel more comfortable than I do. Her relaxed attitude changes a bit, however, once our acquaintance enters the room after an hour. He puts on his white coat and invites us into his small consultation room, which is separated from this living room only by an old, torn curtain. Laura takes a seat on the only chair in front of a desk, while I install myself on a low wooden bench placed against the mud wall of this small, dark room.

Although we are both acquainted with this doctor, our conversation unfolds in an atmosphere of unease. With her head leaning on her hands, Laura declares that she missed her period. The doctor asks whether she has already done a pregnancy test. Laura takes a small jar filled with urine out of her pink bag and places it in front of the doctor, asking him whether it could be done now. After the transaction of money for the test, which needs to be retrieved from some unknown source in the city by a young male assistant, and more soap opera drama for Laura and me while awaiting his return, Laura's fear is confirmed when the doctor shows us the two blue lines that clearly appear on the urine-drenched strip. He starts to pose several questions about Laura's menstruation, reproductive history, and the moment of conception—as I have heard him do when I accompanied other informants before. He concludes that Laura's pregnancy has attained eight weeks and explains that an interruption will therefore require two phases: one in which the fetal tissue will be purposefully damaged, and one in which curettage will be performed. In between these interventions, Laura will have to go back to Asung and wait for the blood loss to commence and gradually intensify. Laura agrees. She stresses that whatever the proposed treatment is, she will undergo it. After some financial negotiations, a deal is made for at least the first part of the intervention. We are asked to return toward the end of the afternoon, when all the other patients will have left.

And so we do. Laura is immediately asked to undress and to climb on a table. She removes her underwear but keeps her flowered dress on. The doctor opens a wooden window to let in some light and fresh air. Few words are exchanged. The next few minutes are filled with only the sounds of the doctor's metal instruments, the dripping of Laura's blood from the table into a bucket on the sandy floor, and the voices of playing children in the courtyard outside. Laura keeps silent but has her mouth wide open in order to breathe in and out deeply. She covers her face with her left arm. Suddenly a considerable blood clot appears on the table in between Laura's legs. The doctor examines it, removes the speculum from Laura's vagina, and gives her an injection in her upper left leg. He orders her to descend. While she stands in front of me, silently raising her dress to let the doctor clean her genitals and legs, I ask her whether she feels okay. She points toward both sides of her belly: "my fallopian tubes." The doctor does not react; Laura silently puts on her underwear and picks up her pink bag.

Armed with a prescription for antibiotics and clear instructions as to the expected process and the envisaged return for curettage, we leave the room a few minutes later. Laura immediately starts complaining about how this abortion was much more painful than the others she underwent but firmly states that she will endure all pain from now onward. She doubts whether she will go back for the required curettage, especially since financial means are lacking. She does not even have money for sanitary towels and the required antibiotics—which, after our return to the village, appear to be out of stock in the health center anyway. When I visit her in the evening to give her my own sanitary towels and some antibiotics, she immediately takes me inside her mother's dark kitchen where she is preparing a vegetable sauce that will be served with couscous. For a second time today, she lifts her dress in front of me—this time to put a sanitary towel in her underwear on which some first drops of blood are already visible. While pulling up her panties, she whispers with a mixture of doubt and relief, "We will see what will happen now. Since my blood is very strong, it often has difficulties to release. My pregnancies don't fall quickly . . ."

In the days that follow, Laura suffers from constant abdominal pain but loses no blood. Hidden in her dark bedroom in order not to attract people's attention, she is visited only by me and her mother, who offers her indigenous remedies to quicken the "fall of the fetus." The absence of any signs of progress, as well as of any medical follow-up, make me a bit anxious. Aware of the national illegality of such practices and of the local fuss that can erupt when abortions go awry, I suddenly feel strangely complicit and vulnerable myself. The many hours I subsequently spend by Laura's side on her bed are meant not only to offer her some company and distraction, but also to monitor the situation for my own reassurance. Laura stays calm and confident, however. During the long conversations we have in her dark room, she reconsiders the previous abortion attempts she has undertaken, and always shared with me, from the very moment I had met her—some five years before.

Indeed, during my first fieldwork period, the then twenty-one-year-old Laura had told me how she had conceived with Omar, a Muslim from the North of Cameroon, while she followed a sewing training at the Women's Empowerment and Family Center in Bertoua.[9] After having been pursued by Omar for two years, Laura had "fallen in his trap" by accepting his money and cooking for him in exchange. Despite her fear that followed a forced defloration, Laura—encouraged by her friend's words that "it hurts for all women"—had returned to Omar and invested the money she received from him in her education. Not long afterward, she had conceived a pregnancy. Her regrets were deep. Fearing that a pregnancy might interfere with her sewing training, she asked her schoolmates how to get rid of this accident. She used everything she was advised to swallow, insert, or purge: Nivaquine pills, salty water, Nescafé. Nothing helped.

That same month, she left to Asung to spend the holidays with her parents. Leaving a letter to Omar announcing her pregnancy and abortion plans, she continued to take remedies upon her arrival in the village. Her practices were soon detected by her mother mama Denise, who, upon hearing the news of a pregnancy, agreed with her daughter's abortion attempts. "My mother feared the reaction of my father, she didn't like Omar at all, and she wanted me to finish school first," Laura stated. No blood loss was achieved, however, and Laura started to feel ill instead. In the village hospital where her mother took her, her activities were soon discovered and heavily reprimanded by the doctor. "He told me that my blood was dying already and I should stop immediately." He gave her injections to prevent the pregnancy from leaving.

Whether convinced by the doctor's warnings or afraid to reveal her own complicity, mama Denise started to publicly scold her daughter as well. "I told her there is her own body and there is a growing child in her body, and that I didn't want to lose any of these two," mama Denise recalled to me later. She insisted that Laura should keep the pregnancy and give the child to her instead. Since mama Denise herself had only one daughter and two sons, and had experienced three additional reproductive mishaps, she would consider this first grandchild as an extra child for herself. This proposal made

Laura furious; it had gone against all her expectations that her mother had *agreed* with her abortion attempts in the first place—and even more that she now wanted to claim "the child she had refused from the very beginning." Nevertheless, Laura quit her abortion attempts. Next to her mother's change of heart, this decision was inspired by her fear of God and destiny. As she remembered that Pope John Paul II had once said that all aborting women in Cameroon should die, she developed a fear for the wrath of God. "Initially, I had thought that God would understand my situation, but the pope's curse got me scared."[10] Moreover, she realized that the child that she was to abort could be "the only one in her belly" or that all other future children could get upset with her abortion attempts, flee, and never come back. All in all, Laura told me back then, it would be better to just keep the child.

However, she continued to contest mama Denise's proposal—gradually supported by Laura's father and two brothers—that she give this child to her parents. Her argument that she could not leave her child in "la souffrance" of her family's poverty led to the indignation of her father and older brother, who had always borne the burden of financing Laura's training in Bertoua. "We walked barefoot here in the village to send our children to school, and then we were reproached for being poor; it made me very angry, and my eldest son also blamed his sister," Laura's father admitted to me. While the two men stopped their financial contributions to her education, Laura's relationship with mama Denise also rapidly deteriorated "until we even seemed to be co-wives, since we didn't talk to each other anymore."

Fed up with these tensions, the pregnant Laura fled from the village to Bertoua. Omar was furious upon discovering that she had *not* aborted, since he wanted to invest his money in the house he was building, and not in a girl-friend and a child. Laura, in turn, asked him for 25,000 CFA francs (around 38 euros), which she claimed to need for an abortion in a hospital, but which she used for prenatal consultations instead. Omar's discovery of this situation infuriated him even more, and he broke all contact with Laura. She therefore decided to charge a complaint against him. "I had warned him to never underestimate me. I haven't spent my time for nothing in the training center. I learned a lot about women's rights." She declared Omar's neglect to the police, without, however, mentioning a word about the abortion attempts and agreements. The policemen summoned Omar and advised that they try to arrange the affair informally, before resorting to formal procedures or even Omar's imprisonment.

Things were settled in the end; Omar provided for the demanded medication and the layette even before Laura gave birth to her son Stéphane. However, after the return of mother and child to Asung, Omar was quickly out of sight—no visits, no financial contributions. These were also discouraged by Laura's mother, who refused to receive Omar and told him that she was able to take care of her daughter and grandchild by herself. The first years of Stéphane's life were therefore pervaded by familial contestations about his belonging. Trying to circumvent the constant claims her parents laid on her child, Laura moved back and forth between friends and family members. To the great frustration of her parents, she also arranged for a birth certificate that legally established Omar's paternity. Omar, in turn, not only ignored his son but also married a Muslim woman. Finally, with the prospect of marriage with Omar thus being blocked—since Laura strongly refused polygamy—and with the conflict with her parents becoming too intense, Laura decided to leave Stéphane behind with her mother and to move to a nearby city, where she had been offered a job in a tailor shop. She started to concentrate on schooling again—this time aiming for a dye training—which she financed with petty trade activities and the money she received from temporary boyfriends.

In the relationship with Jean, whom she described as "a typical big fish," she conceived again. While Jean seemed willing to recognize paternity, Laura was reluctant to bear another child at this point:

> I thought, "I still love Stéphane's father. If he will come back to take me into marriage, what will he say if he sees me with another pregnancy?" Because I had made this decision in my life that I would only bear children with one man. And what is more, Jean told me he would take my child, but not me. So why would I keep this pregnancy? Two children, without a marriage? Imagine the suffering! So I told the good God, "Pardon me, I want children, but not with this person. Help me make the pregnancy leave." It was quickly done by a doctor in the evening: with a needle, he removed the water and blood that surround the fetus. He cut the cord that links the fetus to my back; the rest would release automatically. This all happened in the dark, with a torch; there was no electricity. I tell you, in that moment I felt that God was really with me. After a week, I started to bleed. I warned my cousin, who was the only one who knew about this. I had told all other people that I suffered from

the women's worm. As my cousin removed my panties, I told her I had
no force anymore, I felt very tired. I squatted. Plop. At nine o'clock in the
evening, it has fallen! In a bucket. Afterward, we went to bury the fetus at
the garbage dump. If you throw it in the toilet where it will rot away, your
childbearing leaves. But at the garbage dump, the wind passes; you will
continue to give birth.

That Laura was indeed able to conceive again was proven after another
year, during my second fieldwork period. I initially found her living in Bélabo
together with her new boyfriend Michel and her son Stéphane—who was
now circulating between Laura, mama Denise, and the childless daughter of
mama Denise's co-wife. When, after some weeks, I coincidentally met her at
the market, she revealed that Michel had publicly hit her and that she had
taken him to court. In the meanwhile, she had gone into a new marriage with
Philippe, from whom she already carried a pregnancy now. When I asked for
her opinion about these sudden changes, she told me that she felt there was
nothing she could do. In fact, this marriage had been arranged by the two
mothers. Philippe's mother, as the sister-in-law of Laura's boss, had spotted
Laura in the tailor shop where she worked. She had kept on telling Laura that
she wanted her as a wife for her son. While Laura's mother had been flattered
by this promise, Laura had taken it as a joke; she did not even know this son
who lived in Yaoundé back then. But one evening, her boss had called her
into the tailor shop and had presented her to Philippe. After a forced conversation, Philippe had convinced Laura to accompany him to his house, as
a proof to his mother that they had really met. Hesitantly, Laura had agreed.
Once inside his house, Philippe had locked her in his bedroom and had told
her he wanted to sleep with her.

I told him I was in my fertile period and I hadn't brought along anything
[i.e., a condom]. He said, "Well, since you're fertile now, I will condemn
you to me just in one moment. Undress!" We started to fight. I ended up
in my underwear. "Take off your bra." I did so. "Take off your panties." I
did so. "Lie down." I refused. He took his belt and threatened to hit me.
He forced me to open my legs. He penetrated me. I told him that he had
raped me now. He said, "Take it as you want. But from today onward,
since I climbed on you, know that you are my wife. And voilà my baby
that you carry in your belly." I told him that I would take some pills [to

evacuate] as soon as I would arrive at home. He refused. I said, "Why wouldn't I abort this? To make a child is a question of agreement. But you do it like this and you want me to keep it? I can't. Anyway, it is not an abortion, because there is not even a pregnancy yet. I just want to take my products to simply evacuate the sperm." He locked me in his house for several days so that I couldn't do that. He told me, "God has written that it is already somebody from the moment of conception. Don't even try."

Laura thus found herself "stuck" with another pregnancy, which led to immediate symptoms in the days that followed. Philippe therefore started to doubt whether the pregnancy was really his. It strengthened Laura's wish to abort this unforeseen, and now also unacknowledged, pregnancy—out of fear of bearing a second child outside of marriage. However, abortion remained out of the question for Philippe and his mother. Since Philippe already had seven daughters but no wife, and since he was the only son of his mother, the two did everything to keep the pregnant Laura and her son Stéphane with them. Their constant supervision, as well as their hasty presentation and pregnancy announcement to Laura's family, not only prevented Laura from aborting the now publicly known pregnancy but also pushed her into marriage with Philippe. This marriage was encouraged by Laura's mother, who told her daughter that a second child should be borne within a marital framework, that Laura should abandon all her informal sexual affairs, and that the willingness of Philippe and his mother to engage was rare to find these days. "This is what I had hoped for in my heart," mama Denise repeatedly admitted to me. Even Laura's father seemed pleased; while he had blamed his daughter for "spoiling her school" during her relationship with Omar, he now told me that "we all know that daughters are there to finally leave into marriage and bear children."

Laura went into marriage. Nevertheless, her pregnancy remained contested and surrounded by the suspicion of her husband and in-laws, who still feared she could have been pregnant before entering the house. This fear culminated when Laura started to experience pregnancy-related illnesses—the treatments of which were supposed to be paid for by Philippe. Anxious about investing financially in what could possibly turn out to be "false fatherhood," Philippe proposed to terminate the pregnancy. Laura refused. She told him that "God has wanted us to keep it, and we will do so." She also reminded him that she might bear the boy that he desperately wanted. And she acknowledged that she herself longed for another child, because Stéphane would soon return to his father. To convince Philippe to engage, Laura finally uttered a curse: if this child was not Philippe's, it would die right after delivery. If it stayed alive, it would prove Philippe's paternity. In response, Philippe—who disappeared to Yaoundé quickly afterward—and his mother did not arrange for a layette but wanted to first await the outcome of the birth. Laura's daughter stayed alive; Philippe's paternity was confirmed. It took him months, however, to send money to his wife and daughter for a trip to Yaoundé—which eventually happened during my last fieldwork period. Although excited about finally leaving her severe mother-in-law behind so as to "go and see the habits" of her husband in the country's capital, Laura also remained ambivalent about the possible outcomes. Her opinion about Philippe was heavily influenced by the extramarital affairs, alcohol abuse, and violent acts he had displayed before his departure:

> I asked him whether the human rights include the right of a man to hit a woman. That doesn't exist! He always claims that the Bible says that the woman is created after the man and that she should therefore endure his whims. But the Bible only says that the woman "accompanies" the man. This means she is not subordinate, but goes with the man out of free will. I tell you, I will see if I like his behavior. If it doesn't please me, I will be gone. I am not dependent on him. I am a tailor, and I have my own income. I can have a future without a man.

Laura's fears proved justified. In the months that followed, I received phone calls from both partners. While Philippe complained to me that Laura had apparently come for "l'aventure" rather than marriage, since she was "walking a lot on the street," Laura confided that she had found Philippe engaged in a relationship with an old, rich woman. Her refusal of this situation had been met with severe violence by Philippe. She now wanted to flee her marriage. While mama Denise—also speaking to Laura on my phone—first advised her daughter to just "take her heart off" and "endure the suffering," she ended up supporting Laura's marriage refusal. After all, Philippe had not only abandoned Laura during and after her pregnancy, but he had also neglected his obligations toward his parents-in-law. Her initial encouragement of Philippe's bride-price transactions and Laura's childbearing within marriage turned into a refusal of quick engagements and support for Laura's contraceptive plans—thus keeping the option of separation open.

Yet, contraception came too late. During the next phone call Laura told me how Philippe, in order to prevent her departure, had forcefully given her another pregnancy, which she desperately wished to abort. "I already tried everything: salt, quinine in whiskey, *kangwa* with lemon, *cytotec* from the hospital; nothing works![11] But I really can't keep a second pregnancy for him. I suffer here, and I am sure he will kill me one day." Mama Denise added that a third child would diminish not only her chances of separation with Philippe, but also those of a marriage with another man. Mother and daughter therefore agreed that, if only Laura managed to flee to the village, I would accompany her to a well-known abortion specialist and get it done.

And so we did, on that chilly morning in August. Lying on her bed in her dark room during the days that follow, Laura thinks back of all these experiences with mixed feelings. Her joy of having successfully fled the marriage with Philippe is mixed with insecurity about her marital future; her joy of having parents who, after all, seem to support her in her current decisions is mixed with resentment about past decisions negatively influenced by them; her joy of having successfully undergone her first abortion intervention is mixed with insecurity about the final "fall of the fetus"; and her joy of having her two children at her side is mixed with insecurity about the moral implications of having aborted others. She tells me that each and every abortion was followed by a fasting period in which she demanded God's pardon. "Even now I tell him I don't refuse to bear children, but it is my current situation that does not allow for a pregnancy. I suffer. So I pray all day long. Sometimes, when I'm really touched, I start to cry."

In the ensuing discussion on divine judgment and life destinations, I ask Laura how she envisages her future. Surprisingly, she states that she would like to end up with the one she loved most: Omar. While her mother still claims that a marriage between the two would be impossible—invoking Omar's "lack of love" for Laura, the birth of a daughter with another man, and her own love for Stéphane, whom she would refuse to give back to his father—Laura's father displays a more positive attitude toward Omar. It creates new hope in Laura, who speculates:

Here, we often say, "You never pluck a mango to leave it behind on the spot." If you pluck a mango, it is to eat it immediately. If you store it or let it fall, you will not find it again. Somebody else who will pass will pick it up and eat it in your place. It is like that with relationships as well. I found other men because Omar had plucked the mango, but let it fall. Others have come and have picked it up. But I know that if destiny has written that I will be together with Stéphane's father, I will end up with him. Some marabouts told me that he still wants to take me as a wife. And he himself says that he will be the one to finally marry me. When he will come and claim Stéphane, he will take me in his house. He predicted that all my other relations will never last. And you know, Omar is the one who deflowered me. So everything he tells me will be realized, since he is now like my father and mother who brought me into this world. It is like a curse. What can I do about it? The only thing I know is that I cannot make the error of becoming pregnant again. Because I took this decision in my life that I don't want to have all my children with different fathers. I would even want to take contraceptive injections and stay calm. But I don't feel like staying in the village with my parents. I feel like going to the younger brother of my mother in Douala. I would like to start a small trade in jewelry or in wrappers there. Even in Ngaoundéré. There, I might meet Stéphane's father [who originates from this city]. Who knows? It is the destiny of God.

It is in this indeterminate situation that I leave Laura behind. A few days later, after my arrival in the Netherlands, she tells me on the phone that, thanks to some injections she received in Asung's hospital, the fetus has finally fallen. She will soon start contraception and take time to see what the future will bring to her. With Stéphane reaching the age for return to his father, she might follow her son and end up in a marriage with Omar. Now that this fetus has fallen, the fallen mango might be picked up again.

* * *

The stories of mama Rosie and Laura could be considered each other's opposites in at least two ways: in terms of the narrated reproductive experiences and in terms of the geographical areas in which they are situated. Current Western thinking often takes these differences as a starting point for theorizing women's agency and suffering. Yet, such theorizations do not reflect the ways in which Gbigbil women manage, talk about, and give direction to their various life contingencies. In looking *beyond* these differences, I will reveal a shared narrative ground on which women draw to make sense of their suffering and decision-making, and to navigate their reproductive conjunctures.

Before delving into those local idioms, however, the next section will outline some dominant understandings of agency and suffering in lay and scientific thinking. I will show how different fertility events and geographical locations are often associated with one or the other, which, in turn, creates a conceptual divide between female victims and agents. This dichotomous thinking is equally present in writings about, and official discourses in, Cameroon—despite the fact that Cameroonian women themselves, at least those in Asung, seem to hold completely different ideas about their "souffrance" and their abilities to exert "politiques" in order to attain their goals. The second part of this chapter will expose these Gbigbil ideas and illuminate how they direct the navigation of different reproductive conjunctures, by women with rural and urban aspirations alike.

Patriarchy and Modernized Mamas: Agency and Suffering Reinterpreted

Infertility and abortion stories like the ones presented above have often been approached as dissimilar events. The reproductive ambitions of women who involuntarily remain childless and of those who voluntarily abort their pregnancies are perceived to be opposite: *wanting* versus *not wanting* children. Psychologists have argued that these different desires result in clearly dissimilar physical and emotional experiences. Some feminists go one step further. They situate these different aspirations in the light of a supposedly dominant patriarchal order that prescribes women to produce offspring, imbues them with a "natural" desire for children, and grants them social status only if they realize this desire through live births and successful motherhood.[12] Women who remain childless would want to adhere to, but be unable to attain, these norms;[13] those who interrupt their pregnancies are perceived as explicitly contesting them.[14] Infertility has thus been interpreted as the ultimate form of (physical, emotional, and social) suffering within patriarchal structures, while abortion is often celebrated as the ultimate form of agency. Many anthropologists, even if they do not explicitly cling to a feminist agenda, have implicitly reiterated this association.[15] Such a conceptual framework divides women into victims and agents respectively.

The stories and experiences of my Gbigbil friends indicate that reproductive aspirations and the desirability of a pregnancy are often changeable and contradicting; to attribute fixed desires to either infertile or aborting women is therefore always problematic. To conceive the one in terms of mere suffering and the other in terms of agency further reduces the complexity that characterizes conjunctures at both ends of the reproductive continuum. This is not to say that Gbigbil women are not embedded in patriarchal systems or gendered power relations; yet, the mere existence of such frameworks and women's divergent reproductive experiences within these frames cannot form the sole basis on which to predict women's ambitions and levels of agency. Matters seem to be much more nuanced. Not only ambitions, but also women's suffering and agency, are in practice often blurred.

Some feminists have rightfully started to question this strict dichotomy between victimization and agency, as well as the essentialist notion of a "shared female experience" defined by some sort of universal patriarchy.[16] These feminists have, like some anthropologists, called for "a more textured and contextual analysis of the interrelationship between women's oppression and acts of resistance in a wider range of women's circumstances" (Schneider 1993: 397). In this chapter, I do not only aim to answer this call. Taking my informants' practical realities and discursive practices as a starting point, I will also scrutinize the assumption that this dichotomy should be understood within, and is actually the result of, some fixed patriarchal order.

There is yet another way in which dominant thinking divides women into victims and agents. Influenced by modernization theories and development thinking, international and academic debates on womanhood in developing countries have come to postulate an important difference between rural and urban women—or women with rural and urban aspirations, for that matter. Urban residence, education, and exposure to modernity are considered key contributors to both the development and the empowerment of non-Western women.[17] For this reason, those residing in the village are generally depicted as poor and powerless sufferers, whereas their urban counterparts have become icons of development, knowledge, and autonomy. Such images are often quickly married with the aforementioned distinction between women as *reproductive* victims and as *reproductive* agents. Women in villages suffer under patriarchal and pronatalist demands, whereas those with more money, knowledge, and power in the city are able to resist those "traditional" schemes and resort to modern methods of contraception or abortion.

Both lines of thought have been applied to the Cameroonian context as well. Over time, a whole body of knowledge and practice—created by scientists, clergy, and governmental and nongovernmental organizations—has contributed to an image of Cameroonian women as (reproductive) sufferers under patriarchy, who could and should be empowered through their acquaintance with modern, urban frames of reference. The earliest anthropological accounts of the eastern region of the country, for instance, never failed to emphasize the existence of male dominance and the resultant exclusion of women in the local communities. Most ethnographic descriptions relate how men's material power and symbolic authority directly resulted from men's positions as household heads and exchangers of wives in a patriarchal system. As men established rights *over* women (and their fertility) through bride-price transfers, the rights *of* women were noted to be virtually absent in these wife-exchanging communities. Invoking local sayings like "a woman has no voice" or "a chicken does not sing in front of a cock," these sources indicated that women were not only considered subordinate to the orders of men, but also excluded from socially acknowledged powerful positions (Balla 1991; de Thé 1970; Laburthe-Tolra 1981; Vincent 1976). Laburthe-Tolra even speaks of an extreme "objectivation" of women, who are

> at most reduced to the state of economic instrument deprived of
> subjective expression. In all circumstances, she first has to shut up,
> to keep silent. Won, sold, lost at a game, hired, lent, deprived of
> every capacity in the juridical sense of the term, not able to possess
> anything, the woman is held at the margins of all domains, without
> any other bond to humanity than the connection more or less held
> with her lineage of origin and the advantages associated with maternity.
> (Laburthe-Tolra 1981: 890, my translation)

In such a context, women would be able to assume subjectivity only as "producers of food and reproducers of people," contributing to men's status with their labor force and childbearing capacities. These sources have consistently portrayed motherhood as highly valued—by patrilinies and, by implication, also by women, who thereby acquired a place and status within this patriarchal order. Not surprisingly, accounts of induced abortions are strikingly absent in these early ethnographies, and infertility—a widespread phenomenon in the region until the late twentieth century—was merely interpreted in terms of social vulnerability and stigmatization.[18] Depictions like these rendered women speechless in a system that grants them "no voice" and portrayed them as victims who suffer the burden of the patriarchal yoke.

Several colonial interventions and postcolonial institutions have taken up, and contributed to, this image with their discourses of empowerment. Historically, Christian missionaries aimed to play a pivotal role in this process. Ever since they arrived in Cameroon in 1890 and reached the East Province in the 1930s, they have been preoccupied not only with conversion to Catholicism but also with the eradication of structural social issues that they deemed incompatible with the Christian dogma, such as local gender relations and marital arrangements. A 1972 diary excerpt of a Dutch Catholic priest who worked in the diocese of Doumé (which, at that time, included Asung) notes the ubiquity of four unacceptable local habits in this domain: premarital sexual relationships and cohabitation; divorce; polygamy; and levirate (widow inheritance).[19] Apart from being incompatible with Christian conceptions of marriage as a sacred, lifelong, and exclusive framework for monogamous sexual relationships, these issues raised moral questions about women's roles and positions in society.

In order to both regulate women's sexual and marital lives, and teach them about their positions vis-à-vis men, the Catholic missionaries created an institution called *sixa*, which became widespread in the southern part of Cameroon from the 1930s onward.[20] Next to its goal of directly linking conversion with monogamous marriage, it aimed to "liberate" women from local male-dominated and "dehumanizing" institutions. Over time, this discourse of Christian emancipation was reiterated by Western anthropologists and their informants alike. On the basis of conversations with Beti women, for instance, Vincent (2001: 56) claims that "the veritable liberation brought by Christianity to women was the new possibility to make themselves heard: Christianity gave voice to women [. . .]. It is Christianity that gave them the dignity of a human person. Their first way to express themselves was refusal."

Recent developments and institutions have further fed the image of women being in need of "liberation" and "empowerment." Over the last three decades, Cameroon has witnessed the creation of a Ministry of Women's Empowerment and Family (MINPROFF);[21] several laws concerning women's rights (with regard to physical integrity, marriage, divorce, or inheritance); educational programs; women's associations and NGOs; and the yearly International Women's Day on the eighth of March. These institutions proclaim a specific focus on women as independent individuals, who should have the same rights and possibilities as their male counterparts. The discourse on women's suffering is, again, one that takes male oppression and female speechlessness as a starting point, and that posits the adoption of urban, modern frameworks as the key strategy to attain autonomy—in reproductive as well as other domains of life.

Yet, this image of female speechlessness is far removed from daily life realities in Cameroon.[22] The life stories of mama Rosie and Laura, as well as those of other Gbigbil women in the previous chapters, show that much more is at stake than the mere rural subordination to, or the urban contestation of, a supposedly dominant patriarchal framework that renders women speechless. When comparing both narratives, portrayals of rural infertility as mere suffering and urban abortion as pure agency become questionable. What, then, can be said about Gbigbil women's reproductive suffering and agency? The following sections will address this question by looking into women's own perceptions of suffering, fate, and decision-making potential—and the ways in which these play a role in their reproductive navigations.

The Paradox of Powerless Portrayals

Utterances of speechlessness and powerlessness are commonplace in Asung.[23] Whatever the topic of conversation, Gbigbil women would often repeat that they have "no mouth to speak with" (*on n'a pas la bouche à parler*) and that they are obliged (*on est obligé*) to do what others demand from them; what else can they do (*on peut faire comment*)? Any outsider might be tempted to comprehend these complaints in terms of male authority and female submissiveness—consistent with earlier ethnographic accounts and modern discourses of empowerment. Women's idioms of powerlessness would then be interpreted as representing their gendered oppression and lack of agency.

A more thorough investigation of practical realities in the village, however, reveals a discrepancy between women's utterances of powerlessness and their relative independence in both the productive and reproductive domains. While land is the property of Gbigbil men (and their lineages) in

Asung, all married women receive their own plot and work on it individually. Although they may cooperate with their husbands or other women in times of economic shortage or field abundance, in general women enjoy practical and economic independence in their roles as producer (cf. Delpech 1985; Geschiere 1985; Goheen 1993, 1996; Vincent 1976). Similar liberties appear in the domain of fertility. The previous chapters have already shown that women have room to manipulate men, exert power, or engage in secret reproductive interventions—despite men's proclaimed control over their wives' fertility. Further, Gbigbil women are not afraid to charge informal or formal complaints against their husbands or to publicly express themselves in village palavers, police stations, or courthouses. Thus, more must be at stake when women portray themselves as powerless and without a voice. How is this paradox to be explained? What do Gbigbil women imply and imagine when they talk about their powerlessness?

Depictions of powerlessness are expressed in multiple ways. At least four discursive themes can be discerned in women's common complaints: suffering, fate, resignation to religious dogma, and submission to patriarchy. First of all, women deploy a widespread, pervasive idiom of suffering (*souffrance*). When commenting on all sorts of negatively experienced life contingencies, but especially their sexual and marital relationships, women never refrain from stressing their souffrance. Rather than correspond to a patriarchal image of women as oppressed inferiors, however, such complaints of speechless suffering paradoxically create a common denominator of womanhood that grants my informants a feeling of female solidarity and even superiority. It is exactly the capacity to suffer that marks them as good women and wives. Perseverance and endurance—both physically (through working in the fields) and emotionally (through "taking the heart off," as mama Denise advised Laura on the phone)—are highly valued traits inculcated in women from a young age onward. The ability to suffer in marriage is a focal point in girls' education and is presented as *strength* rather than *weakness*—something to be proud of as a woman.[24] It proves not only one's capacity to endure, but also the efforts one is willing to make to attain a valued goal.[25]

Yet, this is only part of the story. If women's reinterpretation of suffering as a form of *hidden* strength might still create the impression of their passive compliance with the dominant framework, in practice it becomes also *explicit* and *instrumental* in their daily life navigations. The religious meanings and merits with which Gbigbil women often imbue their complaints about suffering create this possibility for instrumentality. Comparing their ordeals to those undergone by Jesus, many women talk about their souffrance in terms of a cross they have to carry. During a focus group discussion on agency and suffering, Peggy, a nursery teacher at the Catholic missionary station, noted: "People often say that you carry the cross that God has given to you. And you should carry it to the bitter end. You should always endure your suffering. Suffering is a school of wisdom; it is part of life. You should abandon discouragement. You should be strong and perseverant in order to succeed, in order to dominate this suffering."

Others compare themselves with female biblical personages whose suffering figures prominently both in the Holy Scriptures and in the weekly sermons in church. Gbigbil women with reproductive problems, for instance, invoke the fate of the Virgin Mary, who had to sacrifice her son, or the situation of Elisabeth, who remained childless for a long time—challenges that both were strong enough in enduring. Not only do such religious notions of female suffering make the unexpected adversities in their daily and reproductive lives more meaningful and acceptable, but they also endow women with "feelings of moral superiority" (Notermans 1999: 174). The idea that women carry their personal burden or "cross" during life is often complemented with a notion of divine judgment upon death. On Judgment Day, God will reward those who showed persistence in their suffering. Victims during life will turn into victors after death. Religious rhetoric thus adds a moral element to idioms of distress: suffering is an expression not only of shared female strength but also of individual "moral superiority" that will be rewarded in the future.

This moral projection of religious salvation is tactically deployed in women's social relationships, for, while it promises sufferers to be rewarded, it also posits that those who inflict suffering on others will be punished relentlessly. Claims of one's own moral *superiority* imply others' moral *inferiority*, just as claims of one's own victory imply others' defeat. The discourse of divine judgment can thus be used to comment on the bad behavior of the men and women with which one competes in daily life—in polygynous households or in informal relationships, for instance. Mama Rosie's story illustrates this deployment within a polygynous setting. Her invocation of marital and reproductive suffering confirms not only her own strength and worth as a (religious) woman, but also the moral weakness of her (evil) co-wife, who, by inflicting this suffering, is doomed to be severely punished afterward. By strengthening her point through witchcraft accusations, mama Rosie's portrayal of suffering becomes a translation of daily life struggles into supernatural competitions—from which she will eventually emerge as a good winner, and her co-wife from as a bad loser.

Second, instrumental dynamics are at play in women's idioms of *fate* and God's will. As noted in Chapters 2 and 3, women's marital and reproductive life stories are pervaded by an all-encompassing idea of predestination and divine determination. Paradoxically, however, this idea is tactically deployed at moments when it can give appropriate meaning and direction to critical conjunctures in life. The narratives of mama Rosie and Laura show how the idea of marital predestination coexists with explicit management of conjugal situations. While mama Rosie considered Etienne "the man whom God had given to me," she also maintained relationships with different men, gave her pregnancy to another candidate, and explicitly refused marriage with that same Etienne afterward. Likewise, while Laura justified her partner choices as "written by God," she also acknowledged her active sexual and marital search through the metaphor of the fallen mango—which, just like the Gbigbil sayings "you should never throw bones to a dog" or "a woman is like a *menyenge* leaf," touches on the quick (re)entrance of single or divorced women into a new union. The motivation invoked by both women to "go and see" when they entered marriage underlines their imagined possibility of leaving the union if it turns out to be disappointing—a decision that may again be justified through notions of predestination or God's approval afterward.

Intentional interventions in the domain of fertility are similarly justified through ideas of predestination. Mama Rosie repeated that she had put her reproductive outcomes in the "hands of God," while she also actively searched for different treatments, uttered witchcraft accusations against her co-wife, claimed the children of her siblings, and assured her childless future through the (secret) demand of a marriage certificate. Laura started to interpret her pregnancies as being sent by God after her abortion attempts had failed and prospects of bearing a child had become more attractive. Her expression "God has wanted us to keep it, and we will do so" shows how the deployment of passive notions of fate can be as tactical an option as her decisions to take contraceptives, or to alleviate her current or future suffering through abortions.

Third, more specific than notions of divine predestination are the particular biblical passages that are used for explaining circumstances or justifying decisions. Again, the image of powerlessness that such expressions portray covers the pragmatism with which they are selected and deployed. Insightful is the discussion between Philippe and Laura concerning the passage in Genesis 2:18–24—often invoked by my informants—depicting God's creation of a woman out of the rib of a man in order to give him accompaniment. While Philippe used it to justify women's subordination, Laura inverted its sense to a situation of equality where a woman "goes with the man out of free will." Similar tactical interpretations surround the biblical passages that are invoked as justifications for gendered divisions of tasks and responsibilities. The commandment in Genesis 1:28 to "be fruitful and multiply, and fill the earth and subdue it"—repeatedly stressed by missionaries ever since they arrived in the "underpopulated" East Province in the 1930s[26]—is often cited by villagers to support local patrilineal ideals and to remind women of their reproductive duties. Yet, mama Rosie mentioned it to strengthen her witchcraft accusations and Laura contested it by assuming God's understanding of her abortions. Both women claimed to resign themselves to the "word of God" as ultimate truth directing their lives and decisions but interpreted it differently in different situations.

Fourth, just like biblical passages, local patriarchal notions are situationally used as justifications or contestations of certain circumstances. They form a normative framework that is sometimes confirmed and sometimes contested by practical realities. Both Laura and mama Rosie refer to the norm according to which they should marry with one man, endure his whims, and bear children for him—but also recognize the discrepancy with their actual situations. Thus, Laura's repeated claim that she wanted to "bear children with only one man" is more an ideal that she tactically mentioned in the face of discrepant realities than a passive acceptance of an imposed order. Likewise, her referral to the supposed male desire for male offspring appeared only when Philippe proposed to abort the pregnancy that she herself actually wanted. Rather than a fixed starting point informing women's powerlessness and suffering, patriarchal and pronatalist frameworks are idioms that can be as flexibly deployed as idioms of powerlessness and suffering themselves.

Notions of suffering, fate, religious resignation, and patriarchal submission thus contribute to a general portrayal of powerlessness but veil as much as they publicly reveal. They are often more instrumental to women's navigation of reproductive conjunctures than they seem to be obstructive. They give such conjunctures not only meaning, but also direction since they can be turned into justifications for decisions made and (overt or covert) projects pursued—irrespective of what these actually are. This leads to a paradoxical situation: while women portray themselves as powerless, such portrayals are actually empowering, and even a manifestation of women's power itself.

This paradox works in several ways. First, portrayals of powerlessness create room for *tactics*. In the sense given to the word by Michel de Certeau (1984), these tactics allow women, who might not have the power to define and impose dominant frames of reference, to inventively use and reinterpret these very frames in order to pursue their own goals—without upsetting the dominant order. In this way, tactics are "the ingenious ways in which the weak make use of the strong" (xvii). As an "art of the weak" (37), tactical behavior requires constant adaptation and improvisation; people "must constantly manipulate events in order to turn them into "opportunities"" (xix). Gbigbil women's flexible use of dominant discourses about suffering, fate, religious dogma, and patriarchy can be considered tactical because it happens at moments when clinging to the dominant frame allows women to pursue their projects and to justify their explorations of certain horizons. This is not necessarily to say that women *are* weak, however, but that they are best able to deploy these tactics when they *portray* themselves as weak. The portrayal of weakness is a tactic in itself.

Second, these discourses, and especially the complaints about suffering, create a shared self-perception in terms of "superior womanhood." They can therefore function as *hidden transcripts*, a term used by James Scott (1990) to refer to "discourse that takes place 'offstage,' beyond direct observation by powerholders" and that "consists of those offstage speeches, gestures, and practices that confirm, contradict, or inflect what appears in the public transcript" (4). Hidden transcripts designate the room for, and capacity of, subordinates to define their own subversive worldviews that might *challenge* the dominant order, even if they seem to passively comply with the public transcript of domination. Often, a hidden transcript is the complete opposite of what is proclaimed in the public transcript. In the Gbigbil case, the hidden transcript does not consist of notions that differ completely from those in the public transcript of patriarchal domination and female submission; rather, it attaches completely different meanings (allegedly hidden and shared by women only) to this very public script. As a result, statements of powerlessness paradoxically become empowering.

There is also a less hidden way in which portrayals of powerlessness can become a source of challenge and power. This happens when such discourses (especially the ones of suffering and patriarchal submission) become vehicles to *overtly* denounce undesired situations through appeals to official authorities such as the police or court of justice. As shown in Laura's story, idioms of suffering and submission are effective elements of such public charges because the authorities to which women resort employ frameworks of female victimhood that are responsive to such complaints. Based on (inter)national paradigms of women's subordination and the fight for empowerment, such frameworks imbue suffering with completely different connotations than the women themselves do. Yet, again, in making their complaints compatible with the dominant discursive frame that pervades these public spaces—that is, in exploiting the Western public script that is so critical of female suffering—women search to pursue their private projects and even openly challenge the status quo.

Gbigbil women's tactics and hidden, or less hidden, transcripts counter the omnipresent ideas about women's lack of voice in this region. Women not only *have* a voice but also make it *heard* and, through this, are sometimes even in actual power. Idioms of powerlessness thus veil different kinds of agency that are often considered the exact antithesis of powerlessness: having a voice (i.e., using and reinterpreting dominant frames), making one's voice heard (i.e., actually attaining one's goals through such use and interpretation), and having actual power (i.e., being able to challenge the dominant framework and its power holders, through sharing hidden transcripts or charging public complaints). Different situations allow for different forms of agency; sometimes women can only exploit the "cracks" in the dominant framework, while at other times they can challenge it altogether. Women may not always have actual power, then, but they rarely lack a voice.

Gbigbil women are very aware that tactically clinging to passive discourses enables them to realize different goals. It is what they call their "politique," and they are proud of it. While men would tell me that "women are like children" because they can be easily satisfied, women would readily reciprocate this stance toward their male counterparts, saying that they can be easily misled under the veil of suffering or other expressions of powerlessness. Successful exertion of these discursive "politics" requires skills of anticipation of, and adaptation to, social circumstances. Toward the end of a focus group discussion on agency and suffering, Lianne metaphorically concluded:

We shouldn't have constrained visions, but look a bit ahead. A woman should walk like a cat. Because before posing her feet, a cat knows whether it's good or not good to walk where she walks. If there's a mouse, she knows how to walk. If there's no mouse, she knows how to walk. A woman should do the same. She should know where to walk, what to do, with whom to walk, and what to say, in order to attract people who will form her physically and spiritually. Some women spend a hundred years somewhere without being able to change. But there are others who know how to adapt their lives and language right upon their arrival somewhere. It's these women who will succeed.

For Gbigbil women, whose lives are characterized by constant geographical, marital, and social mobility, adaptation and anticipation might long have been a key to their "success." Such skills allow them to successfully move from their own families into those of their husbands, or from rural to urban areas and back, and to navigate the increasingly unstable political, economic, and social "terrains." Given that "contingency contributes significantly to the creation of experiential uncertainty" (Johnson-Hanks 2005: 370), and that women nowadays live within a "routinized state of uncertainty" (376), it is not surprising that they formulate their (different kinds of) agency as "judicious opportunism" (370) at most: rather than rational calculations based on prior intentions or fixed hegemonic frameworks, their "politics" are immediate reactions to the contingent circumstances and power relations they encounter during reproductive and other conjunctures in life.

This is not to say that women always obtain their goals, of course. Especially in periods of contestation, their tactics, hidden transcripts, or more overt maneuvers can work out in negative ways. In uncertain and ambiguous reproductive conjunctures, for instance, portrayals of powerlessness and power are no less uncertain and ambiguous. The following sections will explore how different discourses of decision-making are at play in the specific conjunctures around infertility and abortion.

Infertility: Accusations and Alternative Forms of Agency

Infertility violates patriarchal norms to bear live children for the family of the husband and is on that basis often described by existing literature and my informants as surrounded by suspicion, accusations, and public insults. The Gbigbil word for an infertile person (*kun*) has been translated as "rubbish," "rocky," and "prisoner" in related Beti languages (Guyer 1984; Héritier 1984; Tsala Tsala 1996); an infertile woman might also be called "a woman of nothing" (*munka asumba*), "a sterile thing like you" (*kun yom da we aná*); or she might face questions like "when will you give birth, huh?" (*wibial di e?*), "have you only come to fill the toilet with excrement?" or "who will bury you when you die?" (*abok a wiwa, zá nye opum?*). In a context where female worth is ideally considered in terms of successful motherhood, the burden of childlessness is said to fall largely on women; though many would admit that male infertility exists, they would also state that it remains hidden under public accusations toward women.[27] Such assertions tend to confirm the image of infertile women as passive sufferers of a patriarchal hegemony.

Within this setting, infertile women are often preoccupied with the portrayal of an image of innocence. Hereto, they tactically deploy an etiological repertoire that presents different levels of culpability. Just as in cases of pregnancy interruption (see Chapter 4), the etiological explanations for infertility are multiple and pervaded by ambiguity—always acknowledging the possibility that the childlessness might be intentionally brought about. Although some people would invoke the "wish" or "creation" of God to explain instances of childlessness, others contested such an account on the basis of God's commandment in Genesis 1:28 to "be fruitful and multiply." They rather focused on the circumstances that may have rendered certain women childless. These can be externally imposed, beyond the will or intention of a woman; both firsthand and secondhand accounts of cruel witches destroying the fertility of their co-wives or competitors—as in mama Rosie's story—abound in the village.[28] But very often, sterility is perceived to be caused by childless women themselves: they must have consciously "blocked" their childbearing; their witchcraft must have "eaten" all the fetuses in the uterus; their disobedience must have provoked a curse by family members; or their sins—such as previous abortion attempts—must have led to a punishment by God. For outsiders, the question of intentionality, as well as the distinction between suffering and agency, becomes blurred and contested in cases of infertility.

Idioms of suffering help infertile women to create an image of innocence. They also form justifications to actively search for (indigenous and biomedical) help; a portrayal of innocent suffering might rouse compassion and induce (financial) support from others and thus increase the chances of obtaining infertility treatment (cf. Feldman-Savelsberg, Ndonko, and Yang 2006). As mama Rosie's story showed, multiple healing sources can be consulted at the same time. Popular in the region are methods that are believed to "wash the stomach"—both indigenous medicines and potentially damaging dilation and curettage interventions in the hospital. Other biomedical procedures are rarely used by Gbigbil women. Although infertility is now recognized as a component of reproductive health, and the fight against it is an explicit objective of the 1992 National Population Policy in Cameroon, biomedical infertility care faces problems and limitations on the ground. In Asung, detection of infertility is based on simple tests and speculations, after which patients are referred to provincial hospitals in Bertoua or Ngaoundéré for an ultrasound. Few are the women, however, who, like mama Rosie, actually follow such a biomedical path.[29]

Since the predominant etiology recognizes disruptions in social harmony as important contributors to fertility problems, and the resulting idiom of suffering is essentially *social* in nature, biomedical examinations are often replaced or complemented with healing methods that take these social causations of infertility into account. Healers and marabouts who constructively draw on occult powers are deemed most effective if supernatural forces are suspected to cause the infertility.[30] Women with fertility problems, like mama Rosie, often use the different explanations of different healers instrumentally within the social relations and power differentials at hand.

Violation of the normative framework and the ensuing inventive search for, and use of, explanations constitute just one side of the infertility story, however. Infertile women may also just reinterpret, contest, or ignore the patriarchal, pronatalist framework. They may downplay their lack of biological motherhood in favor of other identifications or sources of status. Mama Rosie, for instance, claimed that respectful womanhood derives much less from one's childbearing capacities than from "the work that you do in front of the people and your husband." Indeed, in practice, barren women often occupy important positions within their marriage and within the village. Mama Rosie's use of modern knowledge, official positions, and traditional forms of authority illustrates this clearly. Gbigbil men seem to confirm that infertile women are able to hold certain positions *despite* or exactly *because of* their childlessness. Mama Rosie's brother-in-law appointed his dynamic sister-in-law as the governor of his quartier, and papa Gerie told me more than once that mama Rosie was not only the wife he loved most, but also his "wife of ambiance"—able to host his guests, to animate gatherings, and to "talk in his place when he is absent" (de Thé 1970: 386).[31] Even if some people—like Laura and her kin—might contest this explicit challenge to the normative order, such contestations can easily be countered with portrayals of suffering and infertile victimhood that logically follow from the same set of norms.

Also, images of infertility-related suffering—based on notions of exclusive biological motherhood—overlook the possibilities for social motherhood through fosterage.[32] The stories of mama Rosie and Laura illustrate that these possibilities are omnipresent in Asung, especially when women remain biologically childless. Mama Rosie vigorously claimed the children of her brothers, gave her own name to newborn babies, and portrayed herself as a "mother of everybody"; Stéphane circulated constantly between Laura and the childless daughter of Laura's maratre. Rather than "precarious solutions in crisis situations, with somewhat 'deviant' connotations" (Alber 2003: 488), these social forms of motherhood are the expression of a widespread notion of belonging in which "the child of your sister is your child," as my informants often told me. Claims on these children may be tactically strengthened by an idiom of suffering; expressions like "when you suffer all alone in the house, you can take the child of your sister to come and help you out" or "when you see the child of your brother suffer, you can always come and take it" are commonplace in the village. The results of my household survey confirm the ease with which children circulate. Almost half of the 286 women responding to the question of whether they cared for children other than their biological offspring did so affirmatively (see Appendix VI).[33]

Fosterage tactics defy not only notions of biological motherhood, but also portrayals of infertility-related suffering caused by an exclusive patriarchal order. Flexible fosterage arrangements might in fact weaken patrilineal ties and virilocal norms (Alber 2003). Widening our focus from narrow, predefined, hierarchical gender relations to relevant social bodies and social interactions in women's daily lives sheds new light on the suffering that would surround infertile women in so-called patriarchal societies. It allows for a critique of the "narrow, distorted and presentist frame of individualized suffering" around infertility (Hunt 2005: 432). Gbigbil women's invocations of suffering are inherently social, and therefore inherently situational and tactical—not *exempt of* but *exemplifying* their agency. The same holds for cases of abortion, as we will see.

Abortion: Prevention and Proof of Suffering

In Cameroon, not only are abortions condemned by local patriarchal and pronatalist discourses; abortion is also considered a criminal offence within the national legal framework (see Chapter 1), as well as a moral offence within Christian churches. Religious authorities consider even the earliest terminations of pregnancies to be instances of murder that violate the right of the unborn to eternal salvation.[34] While on an international level, prochoice movements have countered this strict dogma—even *within* the Catholic Church[35]—such lobby groups are virtually absent in Cameroon. To the contrary, the potential liberalization of abortion that followed Cameroon's adoption of the Maputo protocol in 2006 was heavily contested by religious (especially Catholic) authorities and associations in Douala in 2009.[36]

Despite this environment of multilevel condemnation, induced abortions are widespread in Asung. Of the 223 pregnancy interruptions reported by 172 Gbigbil women in my survey, 11 percent were indicated to be induced (see Appendix VI).[37] Numerous methods were cited: 60 percent of those twenty-five abortions had been provoked with indigenous products or chemical liquids, almost a quarter had been induced through clandestine curettages performed by biomedical staff in hospitals or informal neighborhood offices, one was the consequence of a conscious overdose of biomedical medicines, and most of the other pregnancy interruptions were the result of the insertion of sharp objects or needles into the uterus. Furthermore, many respondents declared taking measures to "prevent a pregnancy from developing" right after sexual intercourse or when detecting a missed period. Many pregnancies are terminated in the discrete period after conception (when one's reproductive potential has been confirmed) rather than a priori prevented through contraceptives (which are feared to permanently impair the reproductive potential).

Numerous circumstances can make a woman decide to abort. Reasons often cited include young age, fear of parents, the desire to complete education or fulfill other aspirations, instability of premarital sexual relationships, nonrecognition of paternity by the partner, difficult economic situations, or, for married and older women, conjugal problems, extramarital pregnancies, health concerns, or birth spacing.[38] Such motivations show that abortion decisions are not necessarily made by autonomous agents acting *against* condemning systems—as celebrated by some feminists—but always situated within sociostructural constraints and horizons. Once examined within reproductive conjunctures, abortion decisions seem to relate much less to (universalist and individualist) condemning discourses than to local idioms of suffering. These idioms of suffering appear in Gbigbil women's abortion narratives in several ways.

First, many abortions ensue from a perceived clash between patriarchal ideals and real-life practices. The patriarchal framework prescribes men to take financial care of their wives who, in turn, bear children for their patriliny. However, as we know now, in practice these reciprocal expectations are often contradicted by conjugal fragility and insecurity. In these circumstances, women might invoke patriarchal ideals and idioms of suffering to justify their abortion practices: as men and their families fail to assume their financial responsibility, suffering women may decide to neglect their prescribed duty of childbearing. Many are the women who repeated Laura's statement, "I want to bear children, but not in this situation." Attention is thus diverted from what is expected from *women* (that is, children) toward the duties normatively prescribed for *men* (that is, the exchange of bride-price payments or at least financial care for their wives and children). My informant Angélique, who aborted her twins out of "anger" against her neglectful husband and in-laws, explained:

> I aborted, because I was very angry with my husband and his parents. My family hasn't eaten anything! So I told myself, "If I conceive another pregnancy, I will suffer a lot." And we were already with two women in the house. Life was not good when I was all alone; how bad will it become when my husband has already two wives? No, I preferred to abort. My mother supported my decision. She has first suffered to bear and raise me. Now I bear my own children already and she suffers again with them. He should really thank her for her efforts. So I told myself and my family, "I will not bear a child anymore before he pays his debt to my parents and treats me better as well."

Angélique links her husband's disrespect of patriarchal obligations directly to her own suffering and that of her family. This suffering, in turn, becomes a socially acknowledged incentive for further decision-making—in this case, inducing an abortion. Gbigbil women terminate their pregnancies not because they want to act *against* patriarchal norms, but precisely because they take these norms as a starting point—a sort of ideal—against which they interpret the encountered realities in terms of suffering. Again, a discourse that supposedly oppresses women is transformed, through the idiom of suffering, into a discourse that enables and entitles them.[39]

Second, aborting women also transform religious dogma from a condemning into a supportive framework. This was made clear to me when I witnessed how my friend Charlotte and her maratre mama Justine were paid a visit by a blind Jehovah's Witness. They politely offered him a seat and interacted with him for a few minutes but only pretended to listen to him afterward; mama Justine continued her cooking, Charlotte started to install her washed clothes in the sun, and both women constantly yelled at children. The preacher departed not long afterward, but not without having left the message that he had probably intended to discuss at length:

> *Preacher*: I would like to talk about abortion today. Abortion is bad. You should know that sexual relationships are blessed by God. With the Grace of God, He will make sure that your sperm and the man's sperm form a child. At the moment your bloods cross, there is already a child. So if you abort, even a few days after sex, you kill a person. It's bad. And not only do you kill that person, but you also kill yourself. Or if you don't die, you will at least suffer a lot.
>
> *Mama Justine*: I would like to ask what to do if you conceive from a man who maltreats you.
>
> *Preacher*: In that case you should keep the child. For whom do you think this child will be?
>
> *Charlotte*: For the two of you, right?
>
> *Preacher*: But especially for the woman. She will profit a lot from her child. So if your husband maltreats you, you should leave him and endure. Because, if you would abort now, who will suffer? For whom is the suffering? For the woman, right?
>
> *Mama Justine*: The pain, indeed! But if I would have an abusive husband and I see I'm over time, I abort it! Why would I keep it? To suffer even more afterward?

This interaction suggests that the social relationships—and their inherent power struggles—in which pregnancies are conceived and contested are far more pertinent to abortion decisions than the condemning normative discourses of Christianity—or law, for that matter. Indeed, *if* women relate to a condemning supernatural force in the face of abortion practices, it is exactly the idiom of social suffering that they invoke. Laura's repeated claim that God would be able to understand her decision to terminate a pregnancy in certain relationships is a case in point. Again, a condemning discourse does not seem to constrain Gbigbil women or make them act *against* it; rather, it is tactically suppressed or reinterpreted in favor of a discourse of social suffering.

But while abortions may be *induced* because of women's discontent with (present or future) suffering, they can also *induce* suffering. As the expressions of the preacher and mama Justine show, this souffrance is mainly considered to be physiological. Far more relevant than legal or religious menaces seem to be the physical risks and damage of abortion practices. According to many Gbigbil people, attempts to "wash the stomach" or to interrupt what is considered a pregnancy could, especially when this is done with intrusive indigenous medicines, "burn the cord of children" or "make the children flee from your belly." It thus endangers a woman's reproductive future—if not her life.[40] In a setting where women's fertility may turn out to be wanted or necessary in the future, any damage purposefully inflicted is heavily frowned on as unwise—a form of "politique" possibly leading to future suffering. Reactions to several cases of abortion-related deaths in Asung tellingly ranged from pity and lamentation of women's marital and reproductive suffering (which must have caused the abortion attempts), to commentaries like "elle n'était pas sage" (she wasn't wise), criticizing the risky reproductive behavior that resulted in suffering and death.

Idioms of such physical postabortum suffering may also be purposefully deployed, especially when the abortion attempt should remain unknown to outsiders. Presenting the abortion as a spontaneous miscarriage and complaining about the concomitant physical suffering diverts attention from questions of culpability. By asserting themselves as sufferers, and therefore "morally good" women without any evil intentions, women contest any negative image that may result from a reproductive interruption and the associated suspicions (cf. Erviti et al. 2004).

Further, as with cases of infertility, idioms of physical suffering can inform, and raise (financial) support for, treatment itineraries. Since induced interruptions are considered to provoke more and heavier blood loss than spontaneous abortions or childbirth, both indigenous and biomedical treatments (such as blood-producing concoctions, vitamin substances, cleaning purges, or anti-inflammatory biomedical injections) are deemed indispensable to replenish the blood reservoir and to prevent further reproductive suffering. Postabortion care—officially included in Cameroon's 2001 Policy and Norms of Reproductive Health Services and aiming to alleviate abortion-related suffering irrespective of underlying causes or intentions—is designed to allow for such "hidden" instances of health seeking. Practically, however, postabortion services are not only limited, but also largely unused by Gbigbil women. The local doctor in Asung admitted:

> Depending on the stage of the abortion, I can treat it. In case of simple contractions, I can try to calm them down. And if the fetus comes out already, I can treat it like a normal delivery. But if the woman bleeds, I have to refer her. Similarly, in terms of postabortion care, I can only offer her some medicines if she doesn't bleed anymore. But it is rare that women come here after their abortions. What often happens is that women ask their husbands for money for treatment because they claim to suffer so much, but put it in their pockets and never come to the hospital.

The doctor went on to cite the case of my informant Géraldine, which I had closely followed. When she had lost her pregnancy of four months, an enormous commotion ensued after she had demanded 5,000 CFA francs (around 7.5 euros) from her husband for postabortion care and alleviation of her suffering. While she claimed to me to have spent this money on cheap medicines from ambulant sellers and "some good food since you should eat well after a miscarriage," others (including the doctor, who had prescribed some medications but never saw Géraldine back for treatment) blamed her for having used her husband's contribution for her own purposes. Her request to me to finance her postabortum curettage was met by the warnings of others that she wanted to "eat" my money, and that she was probably deploying an idiom of pain and suffering to cover the fact that she herself had induced this pregnancy interruption. Indeed, women's complaints about heavy blood loss, abdominal pain, or other forms of suffering after pregnancy interruptions are likely to encounter the suspicions of outsiders, who are always aware of this possible intentional aspect underlying interrupted fertility. Discourses of suffering are important discourses of decision-making.

Thus, suffering and agency relate to each other in complex ways. Contrary to common assumptions, in eastern Cameroon this holds for both infertility and abortion, and for women with rural and urban aspirations alike. No matter their particular reproductive experiences and aspirations, Gbigbil women resort to a "shared narrative groundwork" (Gammeltoft 2006: 595), based on paradoxical portrayals of powerlessness, that allows them to navigate complex conjunctures. Such discourses of decision-making reveal women's own conceptualizations of their capacity to give direction to their reproductive trajectories, to exploit local "habits of pragmatism" (Lock and Kaufert 1997: 2), and to "optimize the occurrence of promising novelties" (Guyer 2005: 379) in order to pursue their personal projects.

Conclusion

TIME TO GO HOME. After fifteen months of fieldwork in Asung, I leave the village with a mixture of sadness and satisfaction, and board a minibus ready to take me and many others on the long and bumpy ride to the capital. In Abong Mbang we make our first stop, which is also the last one in the East Province. Our overcrowded bus immediately attracts a group of young Cameroonian girls who slowly stride alongside its open windows, with doughnuts, banana chips, roasted nuts, and peeled oranges on the plates above their heads. A man sitting next to me buys some peanuts from a young girl, who looks him straight in the eyes before moving on, hissing to attract other customers. I hear how, with a tone of indignation, the man exclaims to his companion: "Did you see how she was making eyes at me? Girls here in the East Province are not children anymore. They know men at the age of eleven. They are ready to seduce men and teach them a lesson in bed. And they want to give birth quickly and abundantly. I tell you!" As we leave the East Province and its sandy roads behind us, I remember how often I was confronted with this image of East Cameroonian women during my study on reproductive interruptions in the area. Despite its long, well-documented history of high infertility, both Cameroonians and ethnographic sources consistently report abundant sexual activity and reproduction in this rain forest region.[1] Motherhood, they claim, is what matters here. With my Gbigbil informants still fresh in mind, I note how this view differs from the stories I heard in Asung. Women's narratives there revealed not only other reproductive experiences, but also an amalgam of alternative aspirations.

As I visited and revisited the village of Asung over a period of five years, I was able to follow my Gbigbil friends through time and discuss the many developments in their reproductive trajectories. Whenever I arrived for a new fieldwork period, children had been born or had died, pregnancies had been conceived or "wasted," and futures had become imagined differently. People's pathways seemed to be constantly changing and entailed many moments of possible redirection that I have called "reproductive conjunctures." These conjunctures were always situated in contexts of unpredictable social inter-actions and changing social structures; they were part of a much larger and continuous spectrum of unexpected happenings that characterizes daily life in this Cameroonian village. Not surprisingly, then, Gbigbil people's stories proved to be enormously dynamic and diverse. Yet, rather than concluding that everything is just variable and contingent, my aim in this book is to try to trace some meaningful patterns in how women make sense of and give direction to their "wasted wombs." What conclusions can we draw about reproductive decision-making and direction-taking on the basis of the stories of Yvette, Sophie, Laura, mama Rosie, and the many others who appear in this book? And how is this reproductive navigation informed by local config-urations of sociality, individuality, and corporeality? This conclusion ventures some answers to these questions.

Navigation Affected: On Intercontingencies and Social Stakes

Pregnancies and their interruptions are social affairs in East Cameroon. The very definition of a pregnancy, its appropriation by others (all with dif-ferent stakes and interests) once it becomes visible, its management, and the perceived causes and consequences of its interruption are all socially constituted—and therefore, at times, also socially contested. A similar soci-ality pervades the fetus as well. Not only are fetal bodies believed to be made up of the essential physical substances (blood and force) of social others, but their contingent development and demise are also subject to social definitions and negotiations. Both pregnant women and their unborn children, then, are deeply embedded in the social fabric of Gbigbil daily life. In our explo-ration of patterns of reproductive navigation in Asung, the question is how this inherent sociality affects women's decision-making and direction-taking around "wasted wombs." How do women's positions in the social fabric shape the options, constraints, and horizons that appear when their reproduction goes awry?

Before delving into this question, it should be noted that reproductive conjunctures always present highly particular convergences of past repro-ductive pathways, existing options and constraints, and future aspirations. They are unique and idiosyncratic durations. To recount all the options and horizons that Gbigbil women can possibly encounter and explore during such conjunctures—themselves multiple and situated in wider, ever-changing historical, political, and economic conditions—would be an endless enterprise. However, all reproductive conjunctures in Asung eventually touch on similar, locally grounded and shared, dilemmas. Broadly, what is at stake is (embracing or rejecting) motherhood and/or wifehood, and (continuing or abandoning) one's pathway toward rural or urban respectability. In other words, women typically make decisions regarding their future reproduction (i.e., trying to conceive again or taking a "rest"), their sexual/marital relationship (i.e., staying with one's partner, going back to one's family, or moving in with another man), and their broader personal trajectories (i.e., clinging to one's formerly imagined future, or switching focus and possibly location altogether).[2]

These decisions, in all their possible variations, are far from deliberate, "free" choices. Women's pathways and projects, and their potential redirection in light of the constraints and horizons brought about by "wasted wombs," are inherently related to several social configurations. These forms of sociality are neither mutually exclusive nor always equally relevant. Yet, taken together, they form an insightful repertoire of significant interrelationships underlying the reproductive navigation of Gbigbil women.

First, a woman's position among her siblings matters. It makes a difference whether a woman is her mother's first or last daughter and whether she has few or many siblings ("from the same womb" and/or "from the same father but different mothers"). First or single daughters are often highly valued for the bride-price they are expected to bring to the family and are therefore most likely to be put on a pathway leading to marriage and childbearing (in order to encourage the in-laws to fulfil their financial obligations). In case of fertility problems, such women often see their relatives—especially their mothers—more implicated in their reproductive and marital affairs. Depending on the situation, they can encourage their daughters to get pregnant again and "endure" the marriage, accept them coming home to take some "rest," or even advise them to abort pregnancies and leave the marriage altogether. The contrast between the influence of Laura's mother and the absence of Sophie's mother illustrates the point.

Second, one's position within a wider body of kin relations matters. It makes a difference whether a woman was born within or outside of a conjugal framework, and whether she grew up in her own patrilineage or among her maternal uncles. Women like Laura who grew up among paternal kin are more likely to be encouraged to achieve motherhood (within or outside of marriage) as their children can be claimed and added to the patriliny in case of unacknowledged paternity or marital disruptions. Women like Yvette who were born outside of a marital union and grew up among their maternal uncles experience less pressure in this respect, as the matriliny generally does not profit from bride-price payments and their daughters' offspring. At the same time, such women also receive less support in case they encounter problems on their marital or reproductive pathways, as we saw in Yvette's case. They may therefore have fewer possibilities to change those pathways when confronted with a critical reproductive conjuncture.

Third, the position of a woman's kin group within wider networks matters. In the current atmosphere of political and economic nepotism, daughters from extended families in which important persons enjoy informal political power or formal employment in the city are better positioned to profit from the established financial and social capital. As was shown in Sophie's story, such daughters are more likely to embark on pathways toward urban respectability from a young age—through schooling or well-off foster parents in the city, for instance. In cases of pregnancy interruption, these women may be less inclined to cling to motherhood and wifehood—and be supported by their family members and other villagers in this deviation from rural respectability (based on the ethics of production and reproduction). They may also enjoy greater access to financial support to pursue alternative, urban ambitions and to seek medical treatment for their fertility interruptions. That this is less the case for women whose relatives occupy a vulnerable or isolated position in the wider community becomes clear if we look at Yvette's story. Backed up only by her maternal grandmother and (to a lesser extent) her mother, both of whom had precarious positions in the compound of their maternal uncles, Yvette did not have the freedom to drastically change her plans and pathways when she was confronted with critical reproductive events. Alternative horizons were simply few and far between.

Fourth, one's position on the marriage market matters. It makes a difference whether a woman has many or few boyfriends and whether her partner(s) is (or are) eager to engage or not. A woman who has multiple partners in both rural and urban zones, like the young mama Rosie, may feel less inclined to accept or pursue marriage and motherhood with one particular partner than women like Yvette who, as a result of social or physical circumstances, occupy a less solid position on the wider marriage market. Multiple partners may offer multiple horizons and thereby create more room for changing pathways, aspirations, and decisions in case of critical reproductive events. Further, the eagerness of one's partner(s) to engage influences one's navigation of reproductive conjunctures. Especially when paternity is acknowledged and financial commitment shown, motherhood and marriage can become immediate priorities informing reproductive decisions. In the absence of signs of commitment, however, alternative pathways and partners may be preferred instead. Faced with the disengagement of their partners, quite a few Gbigbil women mentioned in this book considered the interruption of a pregnancy to be the only way out of unexpected reproductive conjunctures.

Fifth, if already married, one's position within the marriage matters. It makes a difference whether a woman is the first, second, or third wife of her husband and whether she has a good or bad relationship with in-laws and co-wives (if present). The pressure to be a good wife and mother is often greatest for first wives, as a husband and in-laws are generally most eager to see their patriliny expand at the beginning of a marriage. This was certainly the case in Sophie's marriage with Alain. Subsequent wives are often granted a bit more freedom—as seen in Daniel's approval of Yvette's use of female-controlled contraceptives. At the same time, later wives occupy a more competitive and contested position; their fertility events are usually surrounded by more conjugal complications and explicit reconsideration of one's pathways and aspirations. Fights with in-laws and co-wives, often inspired by fertility-related matters, are common reasons to abandon one's marital pathway. The ease with which this is done depends on whether (any part of) the bride-price has been paid. Although instances of divorce after bride-price exchanges are certainly not rare, the transfer of sums of money from the in-laws to one's own family members (who often immediately consume it and would not be able to pay it back in case of divorce) complicates one's decision to abandon a marriage during critical reproductive events.

What does all this mean for our understanding of women's reproductive navigation in eastern Cameroon? Obviously, the different social configurations affect women's reproductive trajectories in different ways: while some are enduring and define which pathways and projects are feasible for women from the outset, others change over time and inspire women's projects at particular moments. Yet, all of them define the *possibilities* and/or *constraints* to women's decision-making in reproductive conjunctures. Reproductive navigation is thus a socially contingent affair, embedded in different forms of sociality and power relationships. And since the influence of relevant others—parents, siblings, partners, in-laws, co-wives, other villagers—in a particular conjuncture depends in turn on *their* life contingencies, *their* previous pathways, and *their* stakes at that moment, I argue that reproductive decisions are *inter*contingent.[3] In other words, life stories intersect; women's navigation never happens independently from the navigations of those around her. The outcomes of reproductive conjunctures are not the predictable result of individual deliberation and design, but the contingent result of the involvement of social others, and of the ways in which women constantly reconfigure their choices in relation to these others.

Yet, all this does not mean that Gbigbil women cannot maneuver and manipulate the social order. In their reproductive navigation, structured sociality is always confronted by equally present notions and expressions of individuality—to which we now turn.

Navigation Asserted: On Individuality and Tacit Tactics

The life stories in this book have shown how Gbigbil women—whatever their background, marital status, social network, or future aspirations—find room to maneuver through complex social situations when striving after their own goals. Women often have clear ideas about what is at stake for them and the desired outcomes of their reproductive conjunctures—even if such ideas are sometimes tactically disguised under an idiom of powerless suffering. Indeed, it is exactly through what I have called the "paradoxical portrayal of powerlessness" that women find individual and inventive ways to assert their interests and try to influence the course of events. Idioms of suffering and submission are (re)interpreted and used in such a way that they allow women not only to comment on the dominant order but also to manipulate it and tactically attain their own (reproductive) goals. Such hidden transcripts are used by women in both urban and rural areas alike, which points to a common narrative drawn on by individuals irrespective of their particular social context. Given the inherent sociality of reproductive navigation, how should we understand these individual tactics?

To start with, notions of individuality are not unheard of in Asung. In fact, they have a long history in this region, where social relations prior to colonization were organized according to principles of separation and resettlement: once individual men attained a certain age and independence, they would leave their kin group to found an autonomous village elsewhere in the rain forest. Even if a central authority beyond the village level was often lacking, constant power struggles within groups were certainly not absent. On the basis of personal talents and characteristics, men attempted to enlarge their group of followers and gain wider power and influence—which could easily be lost to others (see Chapter 1). Social organization was based on what Guyer (1996: 7) has described as a "self-valuation/realization process whereby the singular pathways of personal expertise were competitively/performatively valued and validated." Individuality *mattered* for the attainment of social status and power.

While this self-realization could historically be achieved only by adult men, nowadays it finds its expression in all stages of the Gbigbil life cycle, for men and women alike. The fetus, once it has attained enough force (ngul), is already believed to be an agent with its own wishes, initiatives, and realizations. Newborn children are carefully examined for individual traits; later in life, they are encouraged to exploit their inborn talents to differentiate themselves from others. Women are constantly preoccupied with their personal "force," needed to direct their (reproductive and marital) pathways and to pursue their particular projects. Individual inventions and improvisations are even considered constitutive of good and successful womanhood, as Chapter 5 has shown. Self-realization—and the attendant preoccupation with one's personal pathways—is a historically rooted "social asset" (Guyer 1996: 6) that is highly valued in Asung's contemporary social fabric.

As for the relationship between such particular pathways and social structures, Guyer (1996: 23) has claimed that "to the degree that the creation of a life trajectory is a prominent principle in the social organization of assets, to the same degree will agency and improvisation have structural salience."[4] Indeed, I found Gbigbil women's focus on individual inventions and interventions to be related to some structural configurations that make up their daily lives. First, women's valuation of individuality is a result of their ambiguous positions as women and wives in society. Owing to long-standing virilocal and patrilineal norms, as well as the current disregard of bride-price obligations, not only are women considered "outsiders" in their partners' households, but they are also often moving between multiple, fragile partnerships and their own families. This situation both demands improvisation from women and offers them space for manipulation.

Second, beyond the marital framework, women and men face structural circumstances that require constant individual creativity. The fluid and uncertain "terrains" described in Chapter 1 can be navigated only through individual improvisation. In the present era—when the economic crisis seems never ending, (urban) opportunities are rare and unpredictable, the practice of witchcraft is believed to be omnipresent, and long-standing norms of social interaction are often breached—"horizons" may vanish as quickly as they appear. The mechanism underlying women's navigation of their reproductive conjunctures is therefore one of "judicious opportunism" (Johnson-Hanks 2005)—a matter of pragmatic improvisation rather than following a preestablished, rationalized itinerary. Instead of having clear trajectories in mind, my informants take promising chances.

Perhaps paradoxically, in the inherently *social* domain of reproduction, this improvised decision-making is often an *individual* affair; reproductive options and horizons are explored individually, inventively, and at times also secretly. Indeed, although nothing is more *social* than reproduction—which ensures the continuation of the social order and imbues parents with social status and power—nothing is more *individual* either. As Gbigbil women are considered outsiders to the patrilineage to which their children officially belong, and as the first few months of their pregnancies are shrouded in silence and denial, fertility remains largely in their own hands. It is this very individuality and privacy that offers them a secret space for decision-making—even if these decisions are never "free choices" but informed by social interests and horizons. Through their individual pregnancy interventions, women navigate the complex social world and the multiple social stakes that surround their fertility.

Such interventions are not always the safest ones in a context where access to safe abortions is severely hampered and where reliable contraceptive methods are sometimes difficult to obtain—or to accept, for those who fear such contraceptives to bring about infertility. In pursuing their personal projects within a complex social landscape and within a deficient health care system, women may inadvertently impair their short-term or long-term health. The fact that their reproductive moves often remain hidden from others unfortunately leads to too many cases such as the one of Celestine mentioned at the beginning of this book, ending tragically without anybody knowing what exactly happened. Such extreme consequences of individual reproductive tactics provoke much gossip and criticism among the Gbigbil; they reveal a reality that men would rather remain ignorant of, that too many women can sadly identify with, and that all of them deplore.

But also more generally, individual initiative has been portrayed as a source of tension in eastern Cameroonian communities, which have long been pervaded by clear ethics of sociality and egalitarianism (Copet-Rougier 1987; Geschiere 1982, 1997b, 2003; Geschiere and Konings 1993; Guyer 1996; Laburthe-Tolra 1981). This tension finds its clearest expression in local witchcraft idioms, which allow people to comment on individual forms of accumulation (and other antisocial practices favoring social inequality) that contravene the long-standing norm of equality.[5] To accuse someone of having witchcraft is to insinuate that this person's actions are led by an enormous occult appetite for blood, flesh, and wealth that is detrimental to social stability. Not surprisingly, such accusations easily erupt around Gbigbil reproduction—a domain pervaded by social *and* individual forces—and around its interruption in particular.

That both pregnant women and their social surroundings might possess ivū and harm the developing baby points to the tension between sociality and individuality in reproductive matters. On the one hand, pregnant women's fear for the influence of malevolent witches shows how reproduction is an inherently social affair, possibly endangered by individual competitors in the social world. On the other hand, the many suspicions that surround women whose wombs have gotten "wasted" shows how reproduction is also considered an individual affair, possibly endangered by some hidden antisocial power in one's belly. The many witchcraft stories that appeared in this book should thus be read as reflecting a historically embedded preoccupation with forms of individuality that have long been recognized but also feared—in Gbigbil society in general, and in reproductive matters in particular.

Apart from the ambiguous associations with supernatural forces, "wasted wombs" also induce women to worry about their own natural, bodily force (ngul). These idioms of ngul represent another set of commentaries on the complex interrelationships between individuals and their social surroundings. One's amount of force is considered individually unique and contingent; it is innate and subsequently altered through life experience. Next to constituting an individual's physical strength, ngul denotes one's power to adapt, to make decisions, to alter ambitions, and to navigate unforeseen conjunctures. In this respect, it is directly related to one's agency. At the same time, it reflects one's status within, and interconnection to, the social world. As Chapter 3 has shown, most complaints of "lack of force" come from those who are deprived of a social network or whose social identity as women, wives, or mothers is under threat. Since ngul is directly linked to childbearing, complaints of forcelessness can moreover be critical commentaries on the social norms to give birth, or on the lack of social support and lack of care after delivery or pregnancy interruption. Such portrayals of physical powerlessness can paradoxically create room for individual maneuvering within the very social order that is implicitly denounced. Complaints of forcelessness can be used to justify individual decision-making that runs counter to social norms and expectations. Yvette's firm resolution to resort to birth control pills and abstain from sexual relationships with her husband after her body had grown "old" and "weak" is a case in point. Idioms of force thus form a complex commentary on existing tensions between individual and social affairs; that reproductive experiences invoke preoccupations with ngul shows how fertility forms the ambiguous crux between these two domains.

Illustrating these tensions around fertility interruption, the Gbigbil stories in this book have shown that reproductive decision-making is not simply a matter of *either* structural dependency and social interconnectedness, *or* individual autonomy. It can encompass both; for the Gbigbil, one does not exclude the other. Women can be intrinsically tied to social others and at the same time enact forms of individuality that are rooted in, and even encouraged by, that same social order. It is this very duality that informs the notion of "navigation": it starts from the assumption that "social structures" and "individuals" are not dichotomous, but always dynamically related to each other. Reproductive navigation happens at the intersection of changing landscapes and moving persons. By zooming in on the intricacies of this navigation, as I have done in this book, we can come closer to the everyday lived experiences of women who carry, avoid, and lose pregnancies within the local world that surrounds and constitutes them.

Yet, if *lived experience* is what we want to describe, we need to consider another aspect that is often ignored by this individual-social dialectic: namely, the material body. The following section points out why focusing on the material body is particularly relevant to the study of fertility interruption, and how it enhances our understanding of women's navigation of the conjunctures around these interruptions.

Body Basics: New Understandings of Navigation

To say that reproductive pathways and projects are both *socially affected* and *individually asserted* is to point to the different (inter)personal dynamics that underlie women's navigation of reproductive conjunctures; to say that the tensions between the two are often verbalized in symbolic idioms of metaphysical powers and physical powerlessness is to point to the meanings women give to these (inter)contingencies. But this is not to say that the actual *physical* experiences around fertility are to be discarded in the study of reproductive meanings and management. Even if bodily concerns—like the ones about physical force—constitute social commentaries, bodies also matter *in themselves*. As Margaret Lock (1993a: 136) once stated, "The question of the body requires more than reconciling theory with practice. It brings with it the difficulty of people both having and being bodies."[6]

And these bodies sometimes appear to have a will of their own. Especially when it comes to fertility and its interruptions, they do not always do what is wanted of them. The stories in this book revealed many possible unanticipated situations: in Chapters 2 and 3, Diana and Yvette tried to "prevent a pregnancy from entering" but nevertheless missed their periods repeatedly; Chapters 4 and 5 described how Sophie, Nadine, and Laura attempted to "prevent a pregnancy from developing" but failed as their interventions to interrupt fetal force filling had no effect. The stories of mama Rosie and Yvette showed how both women, while young and desperate for children, were suddenly confronted with bodily states (infertile and "old," respectively) that made any future reproductive success highly unlikely. Bodies like the ones of Yvette and Celestine unexpectedly collapsed during deliveries or after pregnancy interruptions that turned out to be more "complicated" than anticipated. Such physical signs and surprises affect the meanings women attach to their bodies and the fertility-related projects they pursue in their lives. Reproductive decision-making is therefore possible or constrained not only because *others* act, but also because *bodies* act.

Such an acknowledgment asks for an even more comprehensive understanding of reproductive navigation—one that adds the primacy and praxis of the body (or "body basics") to the individual-social dialectic discussed above. The body does not only enable or constrain women's navigation, but it needs to be navigated *itself* as well; it both *directs* and *demands* navigation. Since acting bodies are unpredictable, women have to constantly manage the broad range of options, outcomes, and obstacles that their bodies present to them. They are confronted with a material world in which anything can happen—the incoherent logics of the body varying between women and over time. Judicious opportunism is thus as much at play at the level of the body as in the uncertain and unpredictable social situations that Gbigbil women encounter.

This bodily navigation—individual and intimate in nature—is always dialectically related to social navigation as women try to align their unpredictable bodies with their social projects. Women constantly supervise, manipulate, and redirect their bodies (and their unexpected workings) in order to successfully navigate the social complexities that make up their reproductive conjunctures. They do so within certain limits, however; methods to redirect bodily workings are neither endless, nor always effective in the face of the body's inherent, and at times persistent, capacity to become pregnant or to release a pregnancy. Nadine's story in Chapter 4 is a case in point: after trying in vain to abort her unexpected pregnancy, which did not fit with her plan to find a rich husband in the city, she used her pregnant state as a potential incentive for three appointed "fathers" to engage—an alternative route into the urban marriage she was aspiring to. By refusing to release the fetus, Nadine's body circumscribed her reproductive navigation; at the same time, this very bodily condition was inventively transformed into a new project on Nadine's pathway to urban respectability. Reproductive navigation, then, is the result of a complex interplay between the body, self, and society.

In this navigational process, bodily processes, personal projects and trajectories, and social situations are possibly redefined. Women's multiple interpretations of physical, individual-intentional, and sociostructural issues question clear-cut distinctions between early and late pregnancy interruptions (Chapter 3), spontaneous and induced abortions (Chapter 4), and suffering and agency (Chapter 5), respectively. The analytical dualities that underlie current thinking on interrupted fertility are much more blurry in everyday practice. The stories in this book have revealed that this very blurriness offers women an ambiguous gray area in which they can pragmatically turn to (partly hidden) possibilities and discourses. "Wasted wombs" can thereby turn into events or be purposefully downplayed as nonevents. All conjunctures around reproductive interruptions can be seen as "socially structured zones of *possibility*" (Johnson-Hanks 2006: 22), because they generate socially structured zones of *ambiguity* that women can pragmatically navigate.

Such a comprehensive view of navigation sheds a new light on reproductive decision-making. It implies that, contrary to the stability that is often attributed to women's fertility desires, reproductive projects change with the hopes and horizons that emanate from women's individual and social bodies. Likewise, reproductive decisions and their outcomes are not fully under women's control, but always inherently related to unpredictable socialities and physicalities. As a result, certain situations are initially *not* chosen but eventually accepted; some choices are *not* made or *impossible* to make despite one's aspirations; certain options are explored but abandoned again; and some outcomes forcibly ensue from the unexpected actions of women's bodies or interactions with other social actors. Reproductive pathways can be strewn with obstacles or lead to hopeful horizons. The directions women take along the way are less a matter of control than the result of a contingent interplay of connectedness, creativity, and corporeality.

Appendixes

Appendix I
Focus Group Sexuality and Motherhood

Today we will discuss the story of Chantal. We will reflect on four particular moments in her life, taking into account five aspects that might play a role at these moments:

- bodily transformations
- transformation of social roles and positions
- daily life experiences
- your mother's advice with regard to this moment
- your own advice to your children with regard to this moment

1. Chantal is the first daughter in her family, living in Asung. She has four younger brothers. Her parents are poor, and Chantal doesn't go to school. She loves to go to the fields, though, and works hard together with her mother. When Chantal is eleven years old, her small breasts start to grow. Her mother takes her *mik* [a wooden stick that is used to prepare the local dish couscous] and starts to massage her daughter's chest. Chantal does not understand why this is done. She continues to work in the fields for another two years. One day, she returns to the village with a basin of water on her head. After storing the water in the house, she starts to do the dishes, as her mother had asked her to do. When she is sitting on the ground, she remarks that her underwear has turned red. She runs behind the house and concludes that there's blood in her underwear. She waits for her mother to return from the fields and explains the problem to her.

2. Chantal's mother advises her daughter to count all her fingers and toes before "knowing" a man [i.e., before initiating sexual relationships]. But since Chantal doesn't have anything to do in the village, some youngsters start to flirt with her and she falls into the trap. A guy takes her to his house when his parents are absent and he asks Chantal to undress. For the very first time in her life, Chantal has sexual intercourse. Afterward, she notices some drops of blood. She is not a virgin anymore.

3. Chantal does now know men very well. But she doesn't know how to protect herself. Since she has never gone to school, she doesn't know how to count her cycle. Her village friends have shown her indigenous remedies that do not seem to work. One day, she waits for her period, but it doesn't come. She waits until she feels a small ball in her belly. She acknowledges that she's already pregnant. Thus, not only is she a woman now, but she will also soon be a mother.

4. Chantal continues to give birth. She bears nine children and has two abortions. Of her nine children, six are still alive; three boys and three girls. These children also start to bear their own children. Chantal even notices that her periods becomes increasingly disordered; sometimes she bleeds twice a month, sometimes it takes three months before it comes again. At a certain point she concludes that her menstruation is over.

Appendix II
Focus Group Pregnancy Interruptions

VIGNETTE 1

Antoinette is a young woman of twenty-two years old. She has one single brother. She just married Antoine, who has presented himself in Antoinette's family with traditional wine. She stays for six months without conceiving, but finally she gets pregnant. She does not tell anybody that she is pregnant. Her pregnancy leaves after two months.

- How will Antoinette and her environment (husband, mother, mother-in-law) react?
- What could possibly have caused this pregnancy interruption?
- What will happen next in this case?

VIGNETTE 2

Bernadette is a mother of thirty-five years old, married with Bernard, who has paid the bride-price for his wife. Bernadette has borne three children: two daughters and one son. The son died, and the daughters have already gone to their marriages. Bernard would still like to have children, and he just took a young co-wife into the household. Immediately, Bernadette conceives. She herself is very happy. After six months, the pregnancy leaves.

- How will Bernadette and her environment (husband, co-wife, father-in-law, older brother) react?
- What could possibly have caused this pregnancy interruption?
- What will happen next in this case?

VIGNETTE 3

Catherine is a thirty-year-old woman, who just lost her husband Jacques. She married him when she was fourteen years old, and in this marriage she got nine children. She often encountered difficulties during childbirth. Two children died just after birth, seven children are alive. Life was hard for the couple, and they had to struggle to nourish all their children and send them to school. When Jacques died, he left his wife with her tenth pregnancy. At the day of birth, the child doesn't want to get out. The case is too difficult for the traditional birth attendant, and Catherine is taken to the hospital. Three hours later, Catherine delivers a stillborn baby.

- How will Catherine and her environment (mother-in-law, sister, traditional birth attendant) react?
- What could possibly have caused this pregnancy interruption?
- What will happen next in this case?

VIGNETTE 4

Désirée is a girl of seventeen years old, who attends secondary school in Asung. At school, she meets a boy from Nkwej [neighboring village] with whom she regularly has sexual intercourse, but both students do still live with their own families. At some point, Désirée doesn't see her period anymore and concludes she must be pregnant. When she tells this to her boyfriend, he denies being the father of the pregnancy, accusing her of having had sexual relationships with others. Désirée starts to cry and tells her story secretly to her friend. Two months after her missed period, Désirée starts to bleed enormously, and her parents have to take her to the hospital. There, it is concluded that she had been pregnant and that the pregnancy has left.

- How will Désirée and her environment (boyfriend, father, mother, friend) react?
- What could possibly have caused this pregnancy interruption?
- What will happen next in this case?

Appendix III
Focus Group Kinship and Marriage

Today we will follow the life course of a hypothetical woman: Charlotte. Just like during the previous focus group discussion, this case is imaginary; Charlotte doesn't exist in reality. But on the basis of her story, we will be able to discuss the different phases of marriage, and their advantages and disadvantages, as well as the relation between her own family and her family-in-law in all cases. Shortly, we will discuss 7 phases in Charlotte's life:

> wangang / engagement > medokh meyal in a faraway village >
> ivoula / bride-price > polygyny > divorce > second marriage
> in her own village > widowhood

Now we will study these phases more deeply by discussing each situation separately. For every phase, we will pretend that we don't know what is to follow in the future life of Charlotte. Let's start zooming in on every single situation.

1. In the first phase Charlotte is still a young girl of sixteen years old. She lives with her own family, but she already fancies village men. She gets pregnant with a guy whom she had known [with whom she had had sexual intercourse], who is called Antoine.
   - What do you think of sexual relationships of young girls before marriage?
   - How did this happen formerly, and what has changed?
   - When is it good to get pregnant before marriage, and when isn't it good?

- What happens between the family of the girl and the family of the guy when the girl conceives?

2. Afterward, Antoine recognizes he is the father of the child. After birth, he brings the medokh meyal and decides to take Charlotte into a village near to Yaoundé, where his family lives. She arrives as a mom in her new family-in-law, the members of whom she has never met before.
   - What will Charlotte's situation become like now? What changes? What do you think of marriages that are this far from the village?
   - When is it good to get pregnant in this initial phase of marriage, and when isn't it good?
   - What happens between the family-in-law and her own family—who are far removed from each other?
   - How do the attitudes of her own family and of the family-in-law (so the maternal and paternal family respectively) change with regard to the children that Charlotte bears in this phase?

3. Time flies. Charlotte bears children. Gradually, Antoine and his family give the kanako, the monni niaŋa bon, and even l'ivoula to the family of Charlotte here in Asung.
   - How will these transactions change Charlotte's situation?
   - How will these transactions affect her desire to bear children?
   - How will the relationship between her own family and her family-in-law change over time?
   - How do the attitudes of her own family and of the family-in-law (so the maternal and paternal family respectively) change with regard to the children that Charlotte bears in this phase?

4. When Antoine has paid all his obligations, he decides to take a second wife into the household. Now Charlotte has arrived at the phase of ival [polygyny]. The second wife also starts bearing children.
   - How does this situation affect Charlotte's childbearing intentions?
   - When is it good to get pregnant in this phase of marriage, and when isn't it good?
   - How will this situation affect Charlotte's position within her family-in-law?

5. After having endured for some time, Charlotte decides to leave her marriage with Antoine. She is thirty years old at this moment. She goes and stays in her own family in Asung. She takes her youngest children with her and leaves the elder ones in the family of her husband.

- What will Charlotte's situation be like within her own family? How will the people in this village view her?
- How will this situation affect the relationship between her family-in-law and her own family?
- How do the attitudes of her own family and of the family-in-law (so the maternal and paternal family respectively), with regard to the children that Charlotte has borne in her first marriage, change at this moment?
- When is it good to get pregnant in this phase of Charlotte's life, and when isn't it good?

6. Staying in her own family now with her youngest children, Charlotte comes to be fancied by a village man called Bertrand. He even proposes to her to come and live with him, here in the same village.
   - What will be the best decision for Charlotte in this case and why?
   - What will her family advise her to do?
   - How could a marriage in her own village be different than a marriage in a faraway village? What are the advantages and disadvantages?

7. Charlotte has decided to accept the marriage with Bertrand, and since she is a daughter of Bibakung [one of the village's patrilineages], she goes to stay with her children in Kidong [another patrilineage in the village]. Unfortunately, after two years of marriage, Bertrand dies.
   - What will happen with Charlotte and her children in this situation?
   - What will Charlotte's own family and her new family-in-law in Kidong say?
   - When is it good to get pregnant in this phase of Charlotte's life, and when isn't it good?
   - What kind of advice would you give to Charlotte?

Appendix IV
Focus Group Kinship Roles

Today we will discuss the story of Christel. Christel encounters three situations in her life that demand public judgments. You will play the roles of different people who will be invited to assist these discussions; randomly, you will be assigned the roles of Christel's mother, her maternal uncle (*ngweej*), her niece (mo kal), her paternal uncle, her father-in-law, her paternal aunt, her grandmother, her sister-in-law, and her boyfriend Paul. From these points of view, you will reflect on the following three situations:

1. Christel is a daughter of the Bibakung family. She lives in this village. Her mother is a daughter of the Kidong family and a mo kal [niece] of the Didabi family. That is, the maternal grandmother of Christel was a daughter of the Didabi family. The mother of this grandmother was a daughter of Bélabo village. She has died already. This woman had a sister in her family [i.e., a classificatory sister] who has also passed away. This sister had gone to Yaoundé during her life and had given birth to one daughter there. This daughter, loose as she was, had conceived a child with an unknown guy in the city. Afterward, she died of AIDS. Thus, her little daughter did not have a mother or grandparents, and she didn't know who her father was. Therefore, she went to discover the place of the maternal uncles of her mother in Bélabo village. During this visit, she knew [i.e., had sexual intercourse with] the father of her child and bore a son, Paul. Afterward, she also died. Paul always stayed with his father in Bélabo and had been raised by his stepmother. When Christel went for commerce to Bélabo's market, she met him. They started a relationship without knowing the connection between their great-grandmothers. When Christel finds herself pregnant, she asks Paul to go and present himself in her family. At that moment, the grandfathers of Bibakung start to trace the kinship of the two persons and detect the situation. They organize a public gathering. A discussion evolves around the question: how to continue?

2. Christel and Paul have understood the advice given to them during the previous discussion. Out of shame, the couple decides not to see each other anymore. Christel stays in her family and Paul returns to Bélabo. In her family, Christel feels ashamed every day. Her ngweejs [i.e., maternal uncles] of Kidong, who pass by every day on their way to their fields, constantly insult her and mock her pregnancy. The shame and anxiety with regard to the future of her child make Christel prefer to abort her pregnancy. Her mother had been informed and had accepted the idea. It is even her mother who searches for indigenous remedies [to abort], but these don't seem to work. Christel is evacuated to the hospital, while bleeding heavily. Here, 50,000 francs are demanded for curettage. Another public gathering is now organized to discuss this situation: what are the opinions of the participants?

3. The gathering has lasted for a long time because of all the discussion points. While everybody was busy talking, Christel died even before curettage could take place. Now the corpse is still in the hospital. In order to transport Christel to the Bibakung family, the corpse will have to pass by the Kidong

family. Everybody now already knows about Christel's case. In the next coming days an enormous discussion evolves before Christel is buried: where will this be, and what are the roles and arguments of each person involved in the discussion?

Appendix V
Survey Questionnaire

Identification number:
Age*:
Date of birth*:
Marital status:

Familial situation

1. Do you live in your own family, in the family of your partner, or elsewhere?
2. Where do your children live?
3. Where do your children sleep?
4. Do you care for children whom you haven't borne yourself? (If yes:) How many? Whose children are they?

Matrimonial situation

5. Has the kanako been paid to your family? (If yes:) When?
6. Has the monni niaŋa bon been paid to your family? (If yes:) When?
7. Has the complete bride-price been paid for you? (If yes:) When?
8. Have you contracted a civil marriage? (If yes:) When?
9. Have you contracted a religious marriage? (If yes:) When?

Pregnancy histories

I would like to talk about all pregnancies that you have had during your life, and whether they have resulted in a live birth or not. A live birth is the birth of a child who cries immediately after delivery.

---

* As the exact age is often unknown or inconsistently reported, respondents were asked both for their (approximate) age and for their (approximate) date of birth.

10. How many live births have you had in your life?
11. Please note for every live birth: What was the child's sex? Is the child still alive? (If yes:) What is the age of the child? (If no:) At what age did the child pass away?
12. How many wasted wombs have you had in your life?
13. Please note for every wasted womb: After how many months of pregnancy did it happen? Was it a provoked abortion or an accident? (If provoked:) How have you provoked the abortion? (If accident:) What was the cause? Which treatment have you searched afterward?
14. Do you know women in your environment who have ever provoked an abortion? (If yes:) How many? How did they do it?
15. Have you ever suffered from the women's worm?
16. Have you ever used remedies after sexual intercourse to prevent a pregnancy from entering? (If yes:) Which remedies?

Appendix VI
Survey Descriptive Statistics

The survey was carried out between November 2007 and February 2008 in Asung and was aimed at reaching the entire female population aged twelve and higher who had had sexual relations. A total of 290 respondents were identified and successfully interviewed face to face. The tables below present the descriptive statistics for the main variables of the survey. The number of valid responses (N) fluctuated considerably from question to question.

Age

Mean	St. dev.	Min.	Max.	N
35.08	16.58	12	83	287

Marital status

Married	Not married	Widowed	Divorced	N
60%	29.7%	9%	1.4%	290

Marital situation

	Yes	No	N
Transfer of kanako payments for (previously) married respondents	47.4%	52.6%	230
Transfer of monni niaŋa bon payment for (previously) married respondents	39%	61%	228
Transfer of complete bride-price payments for (previously) married respondents	30.8%	69.2%	227
Civil marriage contracted by (previously) married respondents	24.8%	75.2%	226
Religious marriage contracted by (previously) married respondents	9.5%	90.5%	221

Residence of respondent

Own family	Partner's family	Other	N
33.2%	63.6%	3.2%	280

Residence of respondent's children

Mother	Father	Both parents	Maternal family	Paternal family	Other relatives	Other	N
14.7%	9.5%	30.3%	14.7%	22.1%	2.6%	6.1%	231

Presence of nonbiological children fostered by respondents

Yes	No	N
48.6%	51.4%	286

Biological parents of children fostered by respondent

Brother or sister	Brother- or sister-in- law	Husband	Son or daughter	Co-wife	Mother or father	Other	N
40.4%	11%	14.4%	23.3%	2.1%	4.1%	4.8%	146

Number of children fostered by respondent

1	2	3	4	5	6	7	8	10	15	N
32.8%	22.7%	18.5%	7.6%	6.7%	5%	2.5%	1.7%	0.8%	1.7%	231

RESPONDENT'S REPRODUCTIVE HISTORY

Number of live births

Mean	St. dev.	Min.	Max.	N
4.11	3.16	0	14	262

Sex division of all live-born children*

Male	Female	N
50.4%	49.6%	245

Survival of all live-born children*

Still alive	Deceased	N
75.7%	24.3%	245

Number of "wasted pregnancies"

Mean	St. dev.	Min.	Max.	N
0.93	1.05	0	5	240

Intentionality behind "wasted pregnancies"

Provoked	Accident	N
11.2%	88.8%	223

Number of gestational months after which respondents' pregnancies were "wasted"

Mean	St. dev.	Min.	Max.	N
4	2.42	1	9	220

Abortion methods used by aborting respondents

Hospital/medical doctor/curettage	6
Indigenous (purging barks or chemical liquids)	15
Drinking concoction of pills	1
Vaginal insertion/needle/opening of cervix	3
N	25

Reasons for accidental pregnancy interruption

Hard work	22.1%
Disease (jaundice, hot water)	48.7%
Women's worm	7.8%
Physical shocks	7.8%
Difficult or premature birth	4.5%
Mystical	1.9%
Other	7.1%
N	154

Kind of treatment sought after a "wasted pregnancy"

Hospital	Indigenous	Nothing	Other	N
49.7%	36.4%	12.1%	1.7%	173

Acquaintance with aborting women

Yes	No	N
31.6%	68.4%	288

Personal experience with "women's worm"

Yes	No	N
47.9%	52.1%	288

**Use of postcoital remedies
to prevent pregnancy**

Yes	No	N
9.7%	90.3%	289

*The total population of respondents' children (still alive or deceased) was 1,077.

Appendix VII
Prohibitions during Pregnancy

Underlying rationale	To protect	Prohibition: "A pregnant woman should not . . ."	Consequence if not adhered to
(Ethno) physiology	Pregnancy	Use remedies for catching fish	Miscarriage since the poison kills the child
		Work in the sun too much	Miscarriage as a consequence of the heat on a woman's back
		Carry heavy baggage	Miscarriage or stillbirth in case the woman falls
		Wear high heels	Miscarriage in case the woman falls
	Delivery	Have sexual intercourse with men other than the father of the child	Difficult childbirth since the woman has "mixed the pregnancy" (elle a mélangé la grossesse; apula abum mon njo) and the child refuses all sperm other than his father's. The woman should first confess by publicly announcing all the names of her lovers before the child can be born.
		Sit with closed legs	Difficult childbirth since the child might not find the opening in the vagina
	Newborn baby	Be woken up when she is sleeping	Malformed child (lacking a finger, an ear, etc.) since the process of development of the child has been interrupted during sleep

(continued)

Underlying rationale	To protect	Prohibition: "A pregnant woman should not . . ."	Consequence if not adhered to
(Ethno) physiology	Newborn baby	Sit down too abruptly (toward end of pregnancy)	Damage of the child's still very delicate head
		Wear tight clothes	Malformed child since there is too much pressure on the belly and the child is not able to develop or breathe properly
		Have sexual intercourse toward the end of her pregnancy (from 7 months onward)	The child will be born covered in a white mucus, with lesions on his body, or with "dirt" in the eyes because of the excess sperm
	Pregnant woman	Wear somebody else's clothes	The woman will catch the same diseases as the proprietor of the clothes
Mother-fetus analogy (physical)	Delivery	Sit cross-legged	Difficult childbirth since the child will also spread his legs when he moves down
		Sleep or rest too much during the day	Difficult childbirth since the child comes out slowly
		Cut her nails	Difficult childbirth since the child cannot scratch his way out
		Wear jewelry	Child will be born with the umbilical cord wrapped around his neck
		Stay in the village without walking to the fields	Difficult childbirth since the child might move into his mother's legs
		Wear a head scarf	Child will be born with the umbilical cord wrapped around his neck
		Stand still in the door opening	Difficult or slow childbirth since the child will get stuck in the vagina

Mother-fetus analogy (physical)	Newborn baby	Chop wood	The child will be born with a split fontanel
		Sleep on her back	The blood of the mother will get into the eyes of the child
Mother-fetus analogy (moral)	Delivery	Quarrel with people	Difficult childbirth since the child will also be angry
	Newborn baby	Steal something	Child will be born as a thief
Food-fetus analogy	Pregnancy	Eat catfish	Miscarriage or the child will be born with a large fontanel that might split at moments of thunder and lightning (ngól)
		Eat fish that has been caught with remedies	Miscarriage since the poison kills the child
	Delivery	Eat the leftover food of the preceding day ("food that has been sleeping overnight")	Child will sleep during delivery and cause prolonged labor
	Newborn baby	Eat alligator	Difficult childbirth since the child will only move upward rather than downward
		Burn meat as a means of conservation	The child will be born with lesions and blisters on his skin, as if he is burnt
		Eat meat that has been partly eaten away by other animals (especially ants)	Child will be born with rash and skin lesions
		Eat the head of a pig	Child will suffer from abscesses on his head

(continued)

Underlying rationale	To protect	Prohibition: "A pregnant woman should not . . ."	Consequence if not adhered to
Food-fetus analogy	Newborn baby	Eat the head of animals	The ears of the child will be filled with pus, and his head will remain very delicate
		Eat an elephant's trunk	Child will be born with a big nose
		Eat snake	Child will crawl only on his stomach, without using hands and feet
		Eat gazelle	Child will suffer from epilepsy
		Eat porcupine	Child will be born with rash, and his skin could tear apart
		Eat turtle	Child will be born as a turtle
		Eat eggs	Child will be born with a bald head and closed eyes; his navel, hands, and feet will swell during life
		Eat certain forest fruits	Child will be born with a tender head
		Eat very hot sauce	Child will burn his mouth
		Eat too much pepper	Child will be born with a long tongue and red eyes, and he will cry a lot
		Eat too much salt	It will swell the woman's hands and feet, and the child will refuse to eat too salty food
Exposure to death	Pregnancy	Walk into a room where somebody has died	Miscarriage or stillbirth
		Assist a funeral without having attached certain remedies to the fingers or hair	Miscarriage or stillbirth

Exposure to death	Newborn baby	Sit down on the bed of a corpse	Child will suffer from "disease of the corpse" (akon mīm) and will swell as if he is malnourished
		Walk on the spot where a corpse has been washed	Child will suffer from "disease of the corpse" (akon mīm) and will swell as if he is malnourished
Exposure to supernatural forces	Pregnancy	Walk alone in the forest too often	Witchcraft attack since the witches might be alerted by the odors of pregnancy
	Newborn baby	Fetch water in the evening	The child will turn mute, since it will be attacked by the witches that had dipped their hands in the water the woman drinks
"Tradition"	Pregnancy	Sit on a bench on which lice are crushed	Miscarriage or stillbirth
		Sit on the skin of a hare (which served as a sheet for newborn babies in former times)	Miscarriage or stillbirth
		Try to kill a snake	Child will get illness mesum with diarrhea and nausea in case the woman fails to kill the snake
	Newborn baby	Eat chicken without her husband	Child will get illness mesum with diarrhea and nausea
		Pass by certain forest fruits	The head of the child will grow explosively

Notes

INTRODUCTION

1. For the sake of confidentiality, I used pseudonyms for all people, all lineages, and most places (except for the bigger cities of Bertoua and Bélabo) mentioned in this book. "Asung" is simply the word for "village" in the local Gbigbil language.

2. Although the word "marabout" can refer to various kinds of traditional healers, my informants use it particularly for Islamic healers from the North of Cameroon, who are believed to "see," and interact with, evil powers or spirits. They can treat both natural and spiritual afflictions through clairvoyance, incantations, and the use of mystical powders or natural products.

3. That moments of pregnancy loss often reveal diverse cultural elements and concerns of anthropological interest has also been acknowledged by Rosanne Cecil (1996), as well as by Linda Layne, who claimed that such moments provide "a powerful lens [. . .] for illuminating many other important dimensions of contemporary culture" (2003: 26).

4. See Rai and Regan (2006) and Regan and Rai (2000). Although the wide-ranging estimates for rates of pregnancy loss may be due to different measuring methods and the fact that many losses occur imperceptibly (Macklon et al. 2002), it should also be stressed that pregnancy loss concerns a biological event that is liable to local variations and frequencies. Thus Margaret Lock's (1993b) notion of "local biologies" may be more relevant than general estimates that either overlook or try to incorporate all local rates of loss.

5. See Bhattacharya et al. (2010), Brigham et al. (1999), Clifford et al. (1997), Heinonen and Kirkinen (2000), and Sharma et al. (2007).

6. I am aware that the word "wasted" can mean many different things in the English language. So does the word "digela" in Gbigbil and the French word "gâté," to which people translate it—with many of their various meanings overlapping. When referring to reproduction, however, the most common signification is the one that denotes destruction: "wasted" takes on the meaning of "spoiled," "ruined," or "ravaged" here. I deliberately maintained the polysemy of both the original word and its French and English translations, as it

213

contributes to understanding the ambiguity and multiplicity of interpretations of reproductive loss in Asung.

7. Recent innovations in reproductive technologies have made this process not only detectable but also visible from a very early stage. The effects of these visualizations on people's perceptions and embodiments of pregnancy, as well as on ideas about the personhood of the fetus, have been documented for different locales (Duden 1993; Gerrits 2016; Inhorn and Birenbaum-Carmeli 2008; Layne 2003; Mitchell 2004; Petchesky 1987; Rapp 2000; Thompson 2005).

8. Some countries take birth weight as an additional criterion for legally separating miscarriages from stillbirths.

9. See, for instance, G. Becker (1994, 2000), Bledsoe (2002), Bledsoe, Banja, and Hill (1998), Boerma and Mgalla (2001), Cecil (1996), Chapman (2010), Feldman-Savelsberg (1999), Gerber-Epstein et al. (2009), Inhorn (1994, 1996, 2003), Inhorn and van Balen (2002), Jenkins and Inhorn (2003), Layne (1997, 2003, 2006), Letherby (1993), Littlewood (1999), Nahar et al. (2000), and Rice (2000).

10. See, for instance, Bleek (1976, 1981), Calvès (2002), de Bruyn (2003), Erviti et al. (2004), Gammeltoft (2003a, 2003b, 2006), Ginsburg (1998), Johnson-Hanks (2002a, 2005), Koster (2003), Nations et al. (1997), Patel (2007), Rylko-Bauer (1996), Renne (1996, 2003, 2006), Schuster (2005, 2010), Svanemyr and Sundby (2007), and Whittaker (2004, 2010). Quite some work has also been done on pregnancy termination after the detection of fetal abnormalities; see Gammeltoft (2010), Rapp (2000), Sandelowski and Jones (1996), and Simpson (2007).

11. Some anthropologists have, however, given the ambiguity of reproductive intentionality its due. See, for instance, the work of Erviti et al. (2004), Kleiner-Bossaller (1993), Koster (2010), Sobo (1993: 254–59), and Whittaker (2004: 112) for references to blurry distinctions between different sorts of pregnancy termination. For discussions on the ambiguous relationship between intended and unintended child deaths, see Scheper-Hughes (1992) and Stasch (2009).

12. For similar arguments, see Cornwall (2007b), Earle (2004), Earle and Letherby (2002, 2007), Jones (2001), and Letherby (1999).

13. See Bledsoe and Scherrer (2007: 48), Grotevant (2007: 123), and Jenkins and Inhorn (2003: 1832).

14. Vigh's work is part of a growing anthropological body of literature on the agency of children and young people. Some of the scholars working in this field have fruitfully placed social navigation and future imaginations at the center of their analysis. See, for instance, Cole (2010), Cole and Durham (2008), and Utas (2005).

15. Conjunctures have been of interest to different social scientific thinkers, for different reasons. Some scholars have conducted "conjunctural analyses" to trace how large structural and historical processes coalesced into particular eventful durations and contributed to their outcomes (Braudel 1980; O'Brien 2000; Sahlins 1985); others—especially sociologists and anthropologists—have attended to the structural specifics of conjunctures in order to highlight the minutiae of decision-making processes (Bourdieu 1977; Johnson-Hanks 2002b, 2005, 2006; Johnson-Hanks et al. 2011; Wagner-Pacifici 2004). Although the particular definitions of "conjunctures" proposed by different scholars vary, what all these approaches have in common is their exploration of the dialectic between structure and action at moments of potential transformation.

16. It is in this way that my understanding of "reproductive conjunctures" differs from apparently similar (and indeed partially overlapping) notions of "biographical disruptions" (Bury 1982), "epiphanies" (Denzin 2001), "critical situations" (Giddens 1979), and "fateful moments" (Giddens 1991), which all imply crisis and eventfulness.

17. What I allude to with this metaphor is, of course, the instance of maternal death. Interestingly, my Gbigbil informants often used the metaphor of "drowning" when talking about maternal mortality—even if this metaphorical drowning was related to an imaginary fall in the water and not to a sinking boat as my whirlpool metaphor suggests (and as was found, for instance, by Jeffery and Jeffery [2010] in India).

18. This flexible, tentative mode of social action has been captured in different terms. Johnson-Hanks (2005: 370) talks about "judicious opportunism," and Whyte (1997, 2002) brings up the term "subjunctivity," while Cornwall (2007a, 2007b) and Lock and Kaufert (1997) propose to see this form of behavior as "tactical" pragmatism. In this book, I am not so much concerned with finding an overarching term, but rather with illustrating how such practices take shape when fertility goes awry.

19. One camp is made up by those who propose a socio-centered view of personhood and selves in African settings (Devisch 1993; Héritier 2003; Lambert and McDonald 2009; Piot 1999; Taylor 1992; Turner 1995); the other consists of scholars arguing that modalities of individualism and potentials for creativity *do* exist in such socio-centered worlds (Jackson and Karp 1990; Nyamnjoh 2002). Also non-Africanists have denounced the dichotomy between a Western ego-centric "individual" and a non-Western sociocentric "dividual." They argue that both individual and social modalities of personhood are present in cultures all over the world, but become variously dominant in different contexts. See Halliburton (2002), LiPuma (1998), Sökefeld (1999), and Spiro (1993).

20. Since the body appeared as a topic of social science research and theorizing in the 1970s, many anthropologists have pointed to its inherent sociality. These anthropologists—ranging from those engaging with the early work of Mauss (1950) and Bourdieu (1977), through those focusing on symbolic representations of society through the body (Boddy 1989; Devisch 1993; Douglas 1966; Feldman-Savelsberg 1999; Godelier 1992; Héritier 2003; Scheper-Hughes and Lock 1987; Taylor 1992), to those foregrounding phenomenological approaches of embodiment since the 1990s (Biehl et al. 2007; Csordas 1990, 1994; Jackson 1998)—have long acknowledged some interrelationship between the individual body and its social surroundings. Some have explicitly deployed the term "social body." Best known for this usage are Douglas (1966), O'Neill (1985), and Scheper-Hughes and Lock (1987)—although each of them has a slightly different understanding of the term.

21. The anthropological methods that I used during fifteen months of fieldwork comprise (in order of importance): participant observation, in-depth interviews (over 250 recorded and transcribed), informal conversations, focus group discussions (twelve recorded and transcribed), body mapping, free listing, pile sorting, severity ranking, village mapping, diary distribution, and two household surveys. These field methods were continuously complemented with archival research in hospitals, the Court of Justice, the Ministry of Health, universities, and various research centers. See Appendixes I to VI for more information about the methods and the gathered results.

22. It was far from easy to arrive at a point where I could roughly understand, and participate in, conversations. As the language had never been officially documented, I had to create my own Dutch-Gbigbil dictionary, as it were, with inventive phonetic transcriptions for unfamiliar sounds and tentative guesses of possible grammatical rules. My interaction with linguists and some archival research at the Summer Institute of Linguistics (SIL) in Yaoundé provided me, to my relief, with some clues about proper transcription methods as well as general linguistic patterns in the East Province.

23. This is, of course, a well-known and debated aspect of retrospective interviews. See, for instance, Rosenthal's (2004, 2006) distinction between narrated life (the life story) and lived-through life (the life history). The understanding and presentation of the self that evolves within the interactive practice of autobiographic narration has been elaborately described by W. Fischer and Goblirsch (2007) and Fischer-Rosenthal (2000), who talk about "biographic structuring," as well as by Rosenthal (2003), who explores the healing effects of this process.

24. My commitment to sound ethical practice transpires in the *ways* in which I say these things: I present the personal stories of my informants in such a

manner that their identities are unrecognizable; I do not use any revealing pictures as supporting visual material; and wherever relevant, I explicitly reflect on my own role in the reproductive conjunctures that I describe.

CHAPTER 1

1. A census conducted by a medical team in February 2014 identified a total of 1,771 inhabitants in Asung.
2. The last Demographic and Health Survey (DHS) from 2011 indicates that the number of inhabitants of the East Province constitutes less than 5 percent of Cameroon's total population.
3. Abega (2007) claims that this massive relocation has had a major impact on sexual and marital practices in the new villages. Contrary to what had happened before, sexual partners could now be selected from lineages that inhabited the same, rather than another, village. This would have led to a decreased control of elders over youngsters, and thereby to a weaker adherence to marital rules and sexual interdictions.
4. The disengagement and mismanagement of the state, the adoption of Structural Adjustment Programs in 1988–1989, the devaluation of raw materials on the international market, and the commercialization of input products had all led to higher costs and lower incomes for Cameroonian farmers. Consequently, the production of coffee decreased from 110,000 tons to 75,000 tons a year, and cocoa production diminished from a yearly 200,000 tons to 120,000 tons in the early 1990s (Konings 1995; Moupou and Akei Mbanga 2008).
5. From February 25 to 29 that year, violent protests took place in Cameroon's biggest cities. The demonstrations followed a strike by transport workers, who were opposing high fuel prices and poor working conditions. Further unrest was related to the generally high cost of living in Cameroon, high unemployment among youths, and President Paul Biya's proposal that the constitution be amended to abolish term limits on the presidency. This would allow him to run in the 2011 elections, despite his long presidency since 1982. Official reports stated that forty people were killed during the riots, but human rights groups claimed that the total must have been closer to a hundred.
6. Plan International has been working in Cameroon since 1996 and is currently active in eleven rural zones in the East Province. In Asung, the NGO constructed a primary school (in 2003) and a kindergarten (in 2008), built wells, connected deprived children (103 in 2008) to foster parents in the Western world, trained traditional midwives, financed medical interventions (mostly related to mother and child health care), organized informative

gatherings on health and social issues, and subsidized the two women's associations, Sol ngon and Seying inĩng, between 2000 and 2004.

7. People in Asung state that there are several forms of witchcraft within the occult world of *mgbəl*, but that *ivũ* is the most important one. Although I heard many contradicting views on the character, origins, and development of *ivũ*, many believed it to be an essentially female and negative form of witchcraft. This inherent link of *ivũ* to the female realm is particularly relevant when fertility problems arise, as we will see in the following chapters. For similar findings and more elaborate analyses of witchcraft in the region, see the work of de Thé (1970), Fisiy and Geschiere (1993), Geschiere (1982), Mallart Guimera (1981), Nyamnjoh (2002), and Vincent (2001).

8. I prefer to speak of "indigenous" rather than "traditional" healers. I do so not only to prevent the much criticized dichotomy between tradition and modernity, but also to reflect the vocabulary Gbigbil people deployed when talking about these healers—who offer treatment "à l'indigène."

9. During my last fieldwork period in 2009, a qualified nurse was appointed who was very eager to improve people's well-being in general and pregnant women's access to the health center in particular. This *dokta* was still present in the village when I finished writing this book in 2016.

10. They are part of the Délégation Sainte Catherine de Sienne of the congregation of Sœurs Dominicaines de la Bienheureuse Imelda, which consists of ten members. The delegation is installed in Bertoua, Kamandjom, and Yaoundé (Bauvineau 2004; Ngo Baleba 2003).

11. Among the information booklets in the waiting room, I found only one leaflet on puberty and sexual behavior. Unwanted pregnancies, induced abortions, and family planning methods were mentioned in overtly negative tones, with a focus on irresponsibility, risks, disorder, and ultimate divine judgment. This official Christian discourse and health policy notwithstanding, one of the local nurses who originated from Kamandjom told me that he informally sells contraceptives at home.

12. This Gbigbil language is part of the Yaoundé-Fang group of languages and falls within Guthrie's linguistic classification A73b (Guthrie 1953: 40).

13. Now that these extended families are forced to live together in one village context, the family elders of these lineages have become political *sous-chefs*. Above these sous-chefs is the *chef du village*, an old man who has occupied this position since 1977 (although officially nominated only in 1994) and lives on a small hill in the center of the village (Sous-préfecture de Bélabo 2007). His status is utterly ambiguous: representing the colonial past and current (failing) state, but at the same time being a family elder of the Bibakung lineage, his actions and expressions are liable to contestation and multiple

interpretations. His particular position is even more precarious since it was his brother who was originally chosen to become the chief.

14. Such a misfortune can be prevented only through the dissolution of the marriage and the performance of a rite called isam. This nightly ritual invokes the "spirit of the forest" (*tĩt isam*) in cases of misfortune, death, or transgressions such as incest and adultery. Initiated men (*ngondj*) sing, dance, and eat around a huge fire and wait for the spirit of the forest to announce itself. With a loud voice, the spirit denounces the culprits of the transgression and demands offerings for the restoration of order. Although there are still some initiates in Asung, gatherings of isam are now officially forbidden as authorities have come to associate the ritual with witchcraft. Similar traditions have been described by Laburthe-Tolra (1981) and Mengue (1982) as *esam* and *sam* respectively.

15. Although the Cameroonian law did first fix a maximum amount of the bride-price, and afterward prohibited the practice altogether, the law remains without effect in reality (Velghe-Scherpereel and van de Wouwer-Leunda 1996).

16. In former times this presentation of the self as a potential marriage candidate for somebody else's daughter—or inversely, the promise of one's daughter to a powerful alliance partner—would often happen without both marriage partners really knowing each other. Rather, marriage would largely be concluded on the initiative of male elders trying to create as many strategic alliances and followers as possible (which makes sense within the "wealth in people" paradigm mentioned earlier). Especially in precolonial and colonial times, when economic hierarchies started to develop, wealthy men had a stronger position in marriage arrangements than the poorer ones. The latter would offer their (often very young) daughters as marriage candidates to the former in order to settle debts or dependencies, or simply to acquire some wealth (Abega 2007). Nowadays, these "child marriages" are absent in the region, although the average age at first marriage in the East of Cameroon is still among the lowest in the country (DHS 2011).

17. The word "kanako" is not of Gbigbil origin but is probably borrowed from the semi-Sudanese Gbaya who live more eastward (Notermans 1999). A proper kanako comprises two goats or two sheep, two knives, two bags of salt, two carboys of wine, two bottles of whisky, two packs of beer, and two glasses.

18. Communauté Financière Africaine (CFA) is a financial community including a number of West African countries that all use the same currency. For purposes of comparison: during my fieldwork, a loaf of bread cost 100 CFA francs (around 0.15 euros). Toward the end of my fieldwork, in 2009, the

national income per capita in Cameroon was 573,372 CFA francs (around 873 euros) per year, or a monthly 47,781 CFA francs (around 73 euros) (see *data.worldbank.org/country/cameroon*). A bride-price thus equals two months of income—which, for villagers without a regular source of revenues, means a considerable strain on their daily budgets.

19. Since 2006 the Cameroonian government has tried to organize and subsidize collective marriages in order to increase the number of legal unions in the country. A news article in the daily *Cameroon Tribune* noted, however, that such interventions often failed because the bride-price, locally perceived as the precursor of a civil marriage, remains mostly unpaid. This article appeared online on June 9, 2011, and was entitled "Collective Marriages: Bride Price Hinders Unions."

20. Legislative provisions stipulate that any surviving spouse should be able to be her deceased husband's successor if he does not leave a direct heir, nor bastard children, nor family members in this position; that she should be able to claim her deceased husband's pension; and that she should have the rights to ask for the division of goods and to be appointed as administrator of these goods while the inheriting children are still minor. Drawbacks are that women have only usufructuary rights on the property that will eventually belong to their children, that they have difficulties effectively administering these goods because of familial pressure and other social factors, and that the division of goods is particularly problematic in polygynous marriages, which are not acknowledged by the French civil code (Velghe-Scherpereel and van de Wouwer-Leunda 1996).

21. This article, written by Brenda Nchewnang-Ngassa, appeared online on November 10, 2013, and is headlined in part "Unlawful Marriage Cohabitation Persists." It describes the stories of two men who are unable to initiate a formal marriage as a result of the high costs of the bride-price and of the formalities around official weddings.

22. This expectation is, however, partly contradicted by a quantitative study on the relationship between premarital childbearing and first marriage chances by Calvès (1999), revealing that the increased chance of marriage pertains only to the very first months after childbearing—and thus probably concerns a union with the father of the child. After a certain time lapse, the association becomes strongly negative; apparently, men other than the father of the child do not necessarily find a woman's premarital childbearing attractive enough to prefer them over single nonmothers.

23. I prefer to speak of kinship as an "idiom" rather than a "system" and thereby stress the negotiability and situationality of kinship norms and categories (cf. Carsten 2004; Franklin and McKinnon 2000; Holy 1996; Strathern 1995).

24. Even before this era, however, mobile sanitary equipments had been formed under the "strategy Jamot" from 1926 onward. Some groups of itinerant health workers aimed to treat patients, protect healthy subjects, and fight against epidemics (especially sleeping sickness). These interventions form the very foundation of public health in Cameroon, called "medicine sociale" at that time (Atangana 1998).

25. In 1968, some efforts were made to improve the national health care coverage through the installation of six experimental DASP zones (zones de Démonstration d'Action en Santé Publique). In these zones, itinerant health personnel started to organize several preventive, curative, and educational activities in the five kilometers surrounding health centers. Although an evaluative report highlighted the receptiveness of the local population to these services, the DASP zones were abandoned in the mid-1970s because of the high costs (borne by the World Health Organization and UNICEF) and the lack of coordination with other interventions of the Ministry of Health (Atangana 1998; Ministère de la Santé Publique Cameroun n.d.; van der Geest 1982b).

26. Medicines would from then on stop being free of charge and being supplied by the Central Pharmacy. Rather, in 1985 a Pharmaceutical Office (ONAPHARM) was created that enabled the sale of essential drugs by doctors. However, the lack of national pharmaceutical policies and the absence of a formal list of essential medicaments have considerably hampered the installation of an efficient system of medical supply and sale (Kamdoum 1994). ONAPHARM was dissolved in 1995, and with the assistance of the German Gesellschaft für Technische Zusammenarbeit (GTZ) and the European Union, a new structure called the National Clearing House for Essential Drugs was created (Wankah, Ndongo, and Abega 1998).

27. The central level is charged with the formulation of health policies and comprises the Ministry of Public Health and health-related research institutes, as well as three General Hospitals and three Central Hospitals. The intermediate level consists of ten Provincial Delegations, their respective Provincial Hospitals, a Special Fund for Health Promotion, and a drug supply center (CAPP). It also has the responsibility of providing technical assistance to the peripheral level. This latter level includes all Integrated Health Centers, offering basic health care, as well as District Hospitals, offering secondary services.

28. The Health Sector Strategy aims to reduce by one-third the morbidity and mortality of the most vulnerable groups; to improve geographic access to sanitary structures offering the "minimum package of care"; and to strengthen management and efficiency at all levels of the health system. The strategy was

updated when a midterm evaluation showed continuing challenges and failures. The revised objectives were aligned with the Millennium Development Goals, and the strategy, initially intended to cover the period 2001–2010, was extended five more years. The main goal of the National Plan of Sanitary Development for 2011–2015 was to support this process of attaining the Millennium Development Goals (Ministère de la Santé Publique Cameroun 2011).

29. In 2014, the Catholic Health Organization (OCASC) had 266 establishments, among which were sixteen hospitals with a total of 3,247 employees. In 2012, the health department of the Council of Protestant Churches (CEPCA), uniting eleven protestant congregations, comprised 180 health institutions, of which there are thirty hospitals (Dimmock et al. 2012).

30. This territorial exploitation and the development of the workforce were realized through the instauration of Zones d'Action Prioritaires Intégrées (ZAPI), financed by the World Bank. Youngsters were trained in the domains of agriculture and community development, and sent to the so-called underpopulated zones, which were to be developed (Geschiere 1982; Ngo Bell 1990).

31. They received monthly family allowances of 1,500 CFA francs per child, prenatal allowances of 9,000 CFA francs, and maternity allowances of 12,000 CFA francs (if the pregnancy could be medically indicated), as well as the reimbursement of one month of salary during maternity leave. Further, taxes would be progressively reduced for those who were married and had children. Benefits would increase until the sixth child (Ngo Bell 1990).

32. The law prohibiting the sale and publicity of contraceptives is no. 29/69 of May 20, 1969, based on a 1920 French law. The regulations with regard to abortion and infanticide are fixed in articles 337 to 340 of the penal law.

33. Law no. 81/10 of July 14, 1980, authorizes the sale of estrogenic contraceptives, but not of condoms. The latter could be obtained only with a medical prescription. In 1990, a new law was created that allowed pharmacists to dispense contraceptives (Ngo Bell 1990; Tantchou and Wilson 2000).

34. Feldman-Savelsberg (2002: 222) has noted, however, that this commission met only once in 1985 and emphasized birth spacing rather than population control as the road to better health and development.

35. The policy covers more issues than only population growth. Its general objectives were: (1) to improve the health condition of the population in general and that of mother and child in particular; (2) to strengthen food self-sufficiency and promote food security; (3) to promote basic education for all, and especially for girls; (4) to develop and promote qualified human resources; (5) to develop and promote the well-being of families and couples; (6) to ensure and promote an integrated and sustainable development of

cities and the countryside; and (7) to promote research in the field of population (Commission Nationale de la Population Cameroun 1993).

36. In order to accelerate the realization of the Millennium Development Goals, the Cameroonian government has been, since 2006, guided by a "consignment note" (*feuille de route*) proposed by the African Union. It aims to circumvent the different defeats observed during the last three decennia (Nsoa Mbondo 2008).

37. Postabortion care comprises five elements: community and service provider partnerships; counseling; treatment; family planning and contraceptive services; and reproductive and other health services (Corbett and Turner 2003).

38. According to this law, every woman who procures or consents to an abortion will be punished with imprisonment from fifteen days to one year, or with a fine ranging from 5,000 to 200,000 CFA francs, or both. The person who performs the abortion on a woman, notwithstanding her consent, is to be punished with imprisonment varying from one to five years and with a fine of from 100,000 to two million CFA francs. These penalties are doubled when the offender engages habitually in abortion, or practices the profession of medicine or an allied profession. In this last case, the court may also order closure of the professional premises and impose a ban on the offender's occupation.

39. Law no. 80/10 of July 14, 1980, stipulates that only pharmacies can sell contraceptives—some of which should be ordered with a doctor's prescription. In practice, the authorization of the partner is often demanded in order to be able to obtain contraceptives, whereas no law prescribes service providers to do so (Beninguissé 2010). Sterilization is accessible only to women of at least thirty-five years of age and who have five or more children. Currently, the East Province is thought to have the largest "unmet contraceptive need" of 32 percent (DHS 2011).

40. In the district of Bertoua (which includes the health area of Asung), only 40 percent of all health centers do actually have a delivery table. Of all pregnant women in this area, 85 percent have received at least one session of antenatal care, and less than half delivered in a medical establishment (DHS 2011).

41. The HIV prevalence rate of 6.3 percent in the East ranks among the highest in the country (DHS 2011).

42. While on a national level about a quarter of all surveyed sexually active women have indicated to have experienced at least one pregnancy interruption, of which 7 percent were induced (DHS 2011), my data from Asung show that 60 percent of all surveyed Gbigbil women have encountered at least one pregnancy interruption, of which 11 percent were stated to be provoked. Nationally, 3.2 percent of all women are estimated to be infertile. In Asung,

6.5 percent of all survey participants indicated having no children, but among them were women of reproductive age who could have borne children later.

CHAPTER 2

1. The situation in which a new pregnancy is conceived while a woman is still nursing a child is called *odangla mon* (you have passed over the child). Not only would it publicize a woman's transgression of the postpartum sexual taboo, but it is also believed to endanger the nursing child's health. The impoverished quality of breast milk, as well as the odors of the new pregnancy, would make the child suffer from diarrhea, nausea, apathy, and, if no remedies are sought, eventual death (see also Fru 2008: 57).

2. Nivaquine is an antimalarial drug based on chloroquine that poses risks of fetal damage during pregnancy. Owing to its availability and affordability in the village, many women use it quite effectively as menstrual regulation or abortion device. This is, however, not without health risks, especially since women prefer to take an overdose so as to provoke a quick interruption of their (possibly developing) pregnancy.

3. Similar ideas about "cords of children" have been expressed by the neighboring Beti in South Cameroon (Laburthe-Tolra 1985) and by women in Gambia (Bledsoe 2002).

4. For comparable findings in other parts of Cameroon, see Aboubakar (2008) and Beninguissé (2003).

5. Similar practices have been described by Eschlimann (1982), Koster (2003), Nations et al. (1997), Newman (1985), Renne (1996), and van de Walle and Renne (2001).

6. Such perceptions about blood seem to be widespread in Cameroon. See also the work of Aboubakar (2008), Beninguissé (2003), Copet-Rougier (1985), and de Lesdain (1998).

7. Gbigbil people often repeat words (in Gbigbil as well as in French) to emphasize the meaning of the word. "Water water" means that a beginning pregnancy contains just some fluids and nothing else.

8. The same could be said about my request to draw gestational processes at one, three, and seven months of pregnancy during the body-mapping sessions. Only later did I realize that such a proposition had been heavily inspired by Western time-based notions, and had probably given women a hard time coming up with a coherent answer.

9. Metaphorical associations of pregnancies with the eating of bananas are widespread in Cameroon. In his book about popular language use in Cameroon, Fouda writes: "With the masculine sex being similar in its form to the fruit of

the banana tree, they say that a girl has swallowed it as they notice that it has stayed in her belly" (Fouda 2004: 79, my translation).

10. Similar dynamics have been found by Aboubakar (2008), Adetunji (1996), Allen (2002), Beninguissé (2003), Chapman (2003), Feldman-Savelsberg (1999), Njikam Savage (1996), and Tsala Tsala (1996), who all stress the *social* and *supernatural* risks to pregnancies and fertility.

11. Next to his duty to attend to all the wishes of his wife or girlfriend, he is not supposed to eat or kill certain bush animals (red hare, porcupine, or snake), or consume certain foods (like chicken or pork) in the absence of his partner. While resorting to sexual activities with other women toward the end of gestation is something that every father-to-be claims to be unavoidable, he should refrain from sharing the bed with others while his partner is giving birth to his baby—lest the latter will be blocked or refuse to be born.

12. In total, I found fifty-one pregnancy-related prohibitions (see also Appendix VII). Some of them have also been mentioned in reports of the Cameroonian Ministry of Public Health (Ministère de la Santé Publique Cameroun 1993b, 1994, 1995) as well as by Beninguissé (2003) and Tsala Tsala (1996).

13. "Vaccinating" remedies means making an incision in the skin and rubbing a mixture of herbal medicines into it. "Evaporation" is done by putting an old pot with boiled cucumber shells and certain remedies under a bamboo bed on which the pregnant woman sits with bare buttocks. The steam of the hot concoction will pass through the openings in the bamboo bed and enter the vagina, where it has a widening effect.

14. A similar attitude toward labor pain has been described by Sargent (1982, 1989). Sargent's analysis of decision-making around birth is comparable to what will be described in this chapter.

15. Ideally, women should not become birth attendants as long as they are still bearing children themselves. Helping women to deliver is believed to block one's own childbearing capacities. In this respect, one woman told me that her husband forbade her to assist a delivery when she was called on for help, since he feared her subsequent infertility. However, as deliveries take many women "by surprise" and need quick intervention, even childbearing women might end up helping their sisters in giving birth.

16. Underwear symbolizes a woman's fertility because of its direct contact with a woman's genitals, her vaginal secretions, and menstrual blood. A grinding pot has been indicated to symbolize the womb by other studies as well (Adetunji 1996; Feldman-Savelsberg 1996, 1999). Similar suspending actions are also described by Taylor (1992) for Rwanda. He calls them poisonous spells that

may not only impede a woman from delivering her baby, but could also prevent her from conceiving again.

17. These massages can be performed in a lying or sitting position. In the latter case, yal sits naked opposite another woman who sprinkles her with cold and very hot water through rapid movements with a wetted traditional broom. Many young women reassure me that the massage, though necessary and effective, is very painful and that they often scream out loud in fear of being burnt. Similar practices have been described by Aboubakar (2008: 67), Beninguissé (2003: 37), and Laburthe-Tolra (1985).

18. As mentioned in the previous chapter, this health center served a total population of 6,049 inhabitants, dispersed over seven villages, in 2014. Around 4,000 people lived within five kilometers from the health center, while more than 2,000 others lived further away. The pregnant population was estimated at 302 women (5 percent of the total population).

19. In contrast to what has been stated by Beninguissé (2003: 19), Gbigbil women did not display a "latent need" to determine the sex of their fetuses. Although some tried to influence the sex of the next child *before* conception—by wearing the underwear or wrapper of a woman who has given birth to many children of that particular sex, or by chewing certain leaves that have a long version (for boys) and a short version (for girls)— I did not hear of any divinatory sessions or indigenous treatments used during pregnancy to determine or influence the sex of the developing child. Likewise, women did not applaud or consult ultrasounds for the specific purpose of knowing the sex of the baby.

20. See Jeffery and Jeffery (2010) for similar findings in a completely different cultural setting.

CHAPTER 3

1. Throughout this book, ellipses, indicating omitted text in quoted matter, are enclosed in brackets, and suspension points reproduced from the originals or indicating trailing off appear without brackets.

2. This choice for modern contraception was inspired by the failures of her previous attempts to prevent conception with indigenous contraceptive methods. Despite burying her menstrual blood in a snail shell, throwing it away on her fields while asking the ancestors not to send her another pregnancy, sending a bottle filled with delivery blood into quickly streaming water, carrying a preventive cord around her waist, and drinking Nivaquine pills and salty water after every intercourse with Daniel, sooner or later Yvette had always found herself pregnant again—a situation she now wanted to avoid at all costs.

3. In case study research, the selection of an "extreme case"—as Yvette's would be termed—is proposed for exploratory research aiming to uncover mechanisms that may also underlie less extreme cases. The extreme case may still be a typical case but just makes common dynamics more explicit. Gerring (2007: 104) notes, "The extreme-case method refers back to a larger sample of cases that lie in the background of the analysis [. . .]. If this population of cases is well understood—through the author's own cross-case analysis, through the work of others, or through common sense—then a researcher may justify the selection of a single case exemplifying an extreme value for within-case analysis."

4. Probably not coincidentally, this is also the place where the spirits of persons mystically killed by a form of witchcraft called *famla* or *mekwain* are believed to go. Here, the poor souls have to work hard on invisible plantations in order to enrich their "owners"—the witches who killed them. About the relation between this spiritual world and babies, one informant said, "Children coming from the world of famla are called *bon mekon*, because *kon* is the Gbigbil word for famla. It concerns people who don't want to work in famla anymore. They say, "I will enter in a new body so that I can be born again." And those children live." That the word *kon* (or *kong*) is used by Beti people to indicate the world of famla is confirmed by Fisiy and Geschiere (1993), Mallart Guimera (1981), and Ngono (2005). Earlier I have mentioned, however, that Gbigbil people also speak of *ayong bekon* to indicate the realm of the dead in general. Clearly, some ambiguity exists regarding the exact provenance of babies.

5. This notion is inspired by Paxson's (2004) discussion of different "ethics of womanhood" in Greece. Paxson sees gender as an ethical "system of virtues," prescribing "what it takes to be good (at being) women or men" (11). She shows how these ethics fundamentally underlie women's sense of self—even affecting what they perceive as their innate "nature." However, rather than a biological destiny, this "nature" should be considered a metaphysical category "in that it requires the social actualization of certain virtues and relationships realized first in practice and second in the public recognition of that practice" (13). That is, only by displaying socially acknowledged virtues can a woman reveal her embodied womanhood, thereby proven to be *good* womanhood.

6. This indistinction is reflected in common funeral rites; whether a fetus dies before, upon, or right after birth, its burial happens in similar ways. Men of the patriliny, especially the woman's brothers-in-law, will wrap the fetus in leaves (*adoli* and *long*), sheets, or a plastic bag and bury it immediately next to the woman's kitchen, often without the mother or other family members being present. On top of the grave, savannah leaves called *long* will be planted

to symbolize the contact between the dead child and this (living) world. This symbol, just like the many words of comfort women may receive from visitors, stresses a quick return of a new pregnancy in the near future. "You have conceived, and you will always continue to conceive" or "a child will always come again" are typical expressions in this respect.

7. Some anthropological studies have revealed similar attitudes regarding the biomedical categories of "miscarriage" and "stillbirth." See the work of Chapman (2003), Earle et al. (2008), Jones (2001), Layne (2003), and Njikam Savage (1996).

8. Menacing pregnancy interruptions are recognized through the warming up of the back, the kidneys, the fallopian tubes, or "the blood inside." Remedies to "calm the belly down" and to prevent the pregnancy from "leaving" include different purges of water with the leaves of *ekol asɔng, noue, molom, abolom*, the bark *mom*, the roots of *abomling*, or the roots of a banana tree. If these interventions do not have an effect, the loss of "water" and "balls of blood" can be accelerated by administering the cooked leaves of an eggplant (*mekei mesong*) or the pulverized leaves of a tree called *adongsi*, mixed with ginger, pepper, and salt.

9. In cases where a woman dies during childbirth without having yet expelled the fetus, a traditional "operation" will be performed on her in the village before she is buried. Under no circumstances is it allowed to bury "two persons in the same grave," lest misfortunes will plague the entire family. In the one case that I witnessed where a pregnant woman *was* buried with her fetus still inside, I was told that male isam initiates would perform some traditions during the night. By making remedies called *nyɔng*, sacrificing certain animals (like white hens, goats, and pigs), and dancing the traditional dance *akong*, they would try to prevent any negative consequences.

10. This moral distinction between mother and baby by Gbigbil informants feeds into the bulk of literature on mother-fetus antagonism (Casper 1998; Hardacre 1999; Heriot 1996; Hubbard 1994; Ivry 2009; Morgan 1996; Petchesky 1987; Rapp 2000), which reacts against phenomenological accounts of intimacy and intercorporeality between a pregnant woman and her baby (see, for instance, Wynn 2002). The critical studies describe how the developments of prenatal technologies, as well as other cultural and historical transformations, have led to a conception of the body, personhood, and rights of a fetus as distinct from and possibly in conflict with those of the mother. Unlike the Gbigbil precedence accorded to a mother's needs and wishes, however, many of these studies show how in Western settings the preponderance of images and rights of the fetus has often downplayed those of the mother.

11. Next to physical treatments, several social conventions are supposed to enhance a quick return of fertility. First, a woman who has experienced a reproductive interruption is not allowed to cry or mourn, since this would prevent a new child from entering her womb. Second, she should have sexual intercourse with the father of the interrupted pregnancy at least once before sleeping with others. This man is thought to have "taken" the woman's fertility, which she can get back only by sleeping with him. Third, no man other than the one who impregnated her is allowed to hit her on the back, lest her childbearing capacities might disappear altogether. These prescriptions once again reveal the tendency to downplay what is lost in favor of what is to come.

12. The first reproductive interruption that happens in a woman's life is often minimized as a matter of "bad luck." Also the death of one or both twins is expected, as these babies are believed to be not only physically vulnerable but also endowed with supernatural forces that may be fatal.

13. The interactions between maternal uncles (*bengweej*) and their sisters' children are often ambiguous, embedded in a joking relationship that allows both parties to claim respect but also to insult or even curse each other (Geschiere 1982; Laburthe-Tolra 1981; Radcliffe-Brown 1940). The ambiguity is reflected in the position of mo kal, which is vulnerable on the one hand (since mo kal is not a direct descendant of the patrilineage) but powerful on the other. Drawing on some uncontestable privileges, mo kal can claim the heads of all animals hunted by mother's brothers, or "speak with force" and kill all the chickens in a maternal uncle's household when it is plagued by conflict or misfortunes. While maternal uncles claim to respect such interventions, they themselves do *not* intervene much in the personal affairs of mo kal—let alone in those of mo kal's children. This explains why Yvette did not consider her bengweej to be a reliable source of support.

14. Much could be said about Yvette's idiom of *suffering* here, but such "portrayals of powerlessness" (and their paradoxical effects) will be discussed extensively in Chapter 5.

CHAPTER 4

1. The story of Sophie's father is quite particular. Having been fostered by his aunt after the death of his parents, when he was ten years old he decided to escape the bad circumstances he had encountered. He offered himself as a servant to a "white man" in Batouri, who eventually sent him to school. With his primary school certificate (CEP), Sophie's father was appointed as a nurse in a hospital in Douala. A few years later, his position changed into that of

a chef de poste agricole in his natal village of Asung. A poste agricole was an institution stemming from French colonial times; its aim was to initiate cocoa and coffee plantations, to distribute knowledge and resources for higher agricultural production, and to "monitor" labor in the fields. The first poste agricole was installed in the ancient village of Ibudim around 1955. After the forced migration in 1967, another post was created in the new village of Asung. It came with abundant territory for the chief of the post, Sophie's father at the time. It is on this territory that he created his own quartier, with his four wives and thirty-six children.

2. As described in Chapter 2, my informants distinguish several forms of women's worms (French: *vers de femmes*; Gbigbil: *song munka*). The "bad" worm that is mentioned here is located in the belly of some women and "eats" all the blood destined to form a fetus after conception. The woman can become pregnant but will eventually miscarry. This worm can be treated only indigenously. The health worker in Asung's dispensary told me that he saw this local conception as an indicator of severe genital tract infections and sexually transmitted diseases.

3. Mectizan (or ivermectin) is used in onchocerciasis and lymphatic filariasis control programs and is freely distributed once a year among the population of Cameroon.

4. The distinction Sophie makes between day and night refers to practices by nonwitches and witches respectively. Witchcraft practices are believed to happen at night and be more powerful or detrimental than attempts to use indigenous medicines by people who do not have any occult powers and only practice "during the day."

5. Sophie's change in fertility desires within the context of this polygynous marriage sheds new light on an age-old demographic debate concerning the impact of polygyny on fertility levels. One camp claims that the competition between co-wives, whose position depends on their reproduction, induces higher fertility levels within polygynous marriages. The other camp counters that the increased level of conflicts, fertility attacks, and marital time-outs would lead polygynous women to bear fewer children during their lifetime. Sophie's story shows that these two hypotheses are not mutually exclusive but that both situations can be encountered within one and the same marriage. Owing to the variability and volatility of polygyny, its impact on the eventual number of children can, at least in eastern Cameroon, not be unequivocally assumed.

6. The idiom of play is highly relevant here for two other reasons. First, Gbigbil people do metaphorically refer to sexual relationships as "play" (see also the discourse of the doctor in Chapter 2). To "play" with a man or woman, aside

from indicating a strategic manipulation of somebody of the other sex, might also simply mean to have sexual intercourse with him or her. Laburthe-Tolra (1981: 510) mentions a similar idiom when he notes that sex is, especially for youngsters, something like "a sexual parade: and they respect the free game, which can only have happy consequences. It is in terms of a play, for that matter, that boys-girls relationships are conceived of. 'Will you begin to play with a girl in the middle of a party without already having played with her in the village?' says the Beti art of flirting." Second, people often describe the inconsistent and flexible lifestyle of youngsters who explore multiple horizons as one in which they "play life" (*jouer la vie*), before starting a serious, settled adult life. Since this chapter will show exactly how sexual and reproductive practices are embedded within wider partner plays and explorations of multiple horizons, I consider the use of the game metaphor extremely appropriate.

7. While this chapter focuses on those who move from the rural area into cities with multiple aspirations in mind, it should not be forgotten that many others move in the opposite direction once their projects become foreclosed. Abega (2007), Akuri et al. (2009), and Lee (1992) have shown that many women who end up as wives and mothers in the village have tried to "search their lives" in cities before. The authors identify illness and deaths in the family, unforeseen pregnancies, arranged marriages, gender discrimination, and poverty as possible obstructions to women's urban opportunities. This is not to say that their aspirations are lost, however; these are often transferred to the children they subsequently bear in the village. In the accounts of my Gbigbil informants, forlorn urban hopes affected not only the future paths of *living* children, but also the interpretations of those who died or were never born.

8. Of course, as Holtedahl (1993: 297) has also noted, ideas about the "good life" in the city are multiple and variable. Depending on their specific stakes and backgrounds, women stress different aspects and advantages of urban residence. However, the specific ideas of each and every one of them fit into the larger framework of easy and honorable city life as sketched in this section.

9. Likewise, Abega (2007: 132) notes for the neighboring Maka that "with money circulating more easily in the city than in the village, and the former invoking a myth of ease, [which is] today well overestimated, youngsters, especially young girls, sometimes try to go and capitalize on their charms there, be it in a temporary manner or in a permanent way." Currently, the idea of a wealthy flow of money in the city is indeed more a "myth" inspiring hopeful action than reality. In practice, salaries—especially those of

women—often remain unpaid for months on end, and many female residents *do* have to work on plots of land in order to reduce food-related expenses. Clearly, the ideals expressed by my informants tell us more about the woes and worries in the village than about the wealth in the city.

10. In this chapter I assume that secondary education is, unlike primary education, most likely to be found in urban zones in Cameroon. It should, however, be noted that since 2007, a secondary school establishment (CES) has been constructed and made functional in the village of Asung, with the help of Gbigbil elites from the Bibakung family. It would be worthwhile investigating to what extent the ambitions and reproductive management of secondary school students who can stay in the village might differ from those who are obliged to move to urban centers and encounter different possibilities there.

11. Whenever I mention the word "modern," I treat it as an emic category. In line with the local meanings and associations of the word, it captures the urban lifestyle and pecuniary honor that my informants aim to achieve.

12. In this respect, Guyer (1996: 13) states that, historically, "triage into those who will be favoured, through education, fosterage and other training, and those who will be gradually sidelined, is a function of *post*-natal social and cultural processes where capabilities and potentials are identified and tracked during the assiduously labour-intensive series of ceremonials and apprenticeships that made up child-raising before the era of schools and world religions." This statement seems applicable to Gbigbil histories as well. Participants of the most important male initiation rite, called isam, were selected by their fathers. Only sons with certain characteristics were deemed capable of undergoing the training and of guarding its secrets afterward. These favored ones were physically marked by incisions in the back of the neck—and are until today proud to show this proof of their selection.

13. With regard to the value of personal characteristics in gaining power within an egalitarian society, Laburthe-Tolra notes, "the possibility remains open to every young, free man, even [if he is] poor in the beginning, to succeed thanks to his dynamism, thanks to his personal talents and capacities [. . .]. The ways in which an adolescent can affirm himself are very diverse: beauty, force, courage, craftiness, intelligence make him eventually worthy of both the favor of young girls, and the esteem of fathers who will be able to "give" him a wife [. . .] because he knows how to hunt or dance well, because he is a champion in fights" (1981: 831–32, my translation).

14. Johnson-Hanks (2007) describes how the concept of "mfan mot" used to denote a certain kind of disposition and honor that was applicable only to *men*. This male honor was linked to material success and dominion over

women; women themselves could not be honorable. The expansion of school, market, church, and state in modern times, however, altered social conditions and cultural schemata in such a way that notions of honor "stretched to include women" as well (645). Johnson-Hanks argues that although this form of female honor is certainly one that derives from the colonial and postcolonial history, it also draws on long-existent notions of honor of the mfan mot.

15. The long-lasting economic crisis and the subsequent delay in bride-price payments are, as noted in Chapter 1, likely to have contributed to this situation as well. Premarital relationships and marital instability are therefore widespread in both urban and rural zones. Yet, as this chapter will show, the ambiguities inhering these partnerships become exacerbated when both partners have other, urban, projects in mind.

16. Interestingly, women in Dakar seem to have a similar way of associating promising male partners with fish; they give those men who offer prosperous prospects the name of an expensive fish, *thiof*. Women even distinguish between small, medium, and big or super thiof according to men's status and potential for generosity (Nyamnjoh 2005). In Cameroon, rich men acting as "sugar daddies" are also been called *cous plies*, meaning "folded necks" (Johnson-Hanks 2006: 173; Meekers and Calvès 1997: 365).

17. This article appeared online on August 17, 2012, and was entitled "Prostitution: Les nouvaux professionels" (Prostitution: The new professionals).

18. This article, written by Pierre Essomba, appeared online on January 26, 2014, and was entitled "Le Minproff fera officialiser collectivement plus de mariages en 2014" (The Ministry of Women's Empowerment and the Family will collectively formalize more marriages in 2014).

19. YouTube is a well-known low-threshold website broadcasting clips, movies, and other videos from all over the world. The reactions displayed here were retrieved on February 11, 2010, from *www.youtube.com/watch?v=oXaQJH-0HSg*.

20. In this sense, men are proud to claim that they are "dangereux"—i.e., that they are popular and successful among the women. Such a public statement is relevant in a context where male desires for sex are naturalized and considered to be a reflection of their biological functioning. In the absence of regular girlfriends, men are liable to become accused of having a "dead penis" (*abin wajaa*)—which poses a serious threat to their masculine identity.

21. The same vocabulary was expressed by the informants of Meekers and Calvès (1997: 365) and Johnson-Hanks (2006: 173). Terms like "ma Meilleure Petite" or "mon Meilleur Petit" coexist with "mon petit" or "ma petite"; "mon copain" or "ma copine"; "mon Chaud" and "ma Chaude"; "Cacao"; "the

Hip"; and "Black Coffee"—all of which aim to distinguish between different sexual partners.

22. See, for instance, the work of Dunkle et al. (2007), Hunter (2002), Leclerc-Madlala (2003), and Nyamnjoh (2005). Their approach has been criticized by Poulin (2007) and Tawfik and Watkins (2007).

23. Not only are pregnant students allowed to go on maternity leave, but they must also be readmitted in case they have been suspended because of their pregnancies, as stipulated by Circular Letter No. 10/A/562/MINEDUC/ESG of January 10, 1980 (UN CEDAW 1999; UN CRC 2000).

24. See, for instance, Basu (2002), Bledsoe, Casterline, et al. (1999), Jejeebhoy (1995), Johnson-Hanks (2006), and Lloyd and Mensch (2008). Many of these studies have investigated the indirect, non-school-related factors that might affect the reproductive decision-making of female students. They argue that the impact of education derives more from the social context in which schooling takes place than from inherent qualities of the schooling itself. This is called the "selection" effect: women who tend to initiate and continue education come from certain socioeconomic strata with particular norms about gender, sexuality, fertility, and appropriate reproductive timing. Further, wider political and economic settings may determine—through mass media, for instance—the use and evaluation of certain educational skills in social practice.

25. *Iwō* is the Gbigbil word for a condition in which a woman's children repeatedly die. Several indigenous treatments of iwō exist, which should all be initiated during pregnancy.

26. Calvès (2000) shows that children conceived within cohabiting unions are approximately six times more likely to be recognized by their biological fathers than those conceived in noncohabiting unions, and that the chances of recognition are four times higher for children whose conception was planned and discussed compared to those whose conception was not anticipated or desired.

27. In 1966, a new marriage law was issued, followed in 1981 by the Civil Status Registration Ordinance. Although bride-price payments were not prohibited by this law, they were dissociated from the legal status of a union. As a consequence, bridewealth no longer determines affiliation or legal paternity.

28. Paternal recognition of children who are not conceived in a legal union usually takes place at the time of birth registration. For such a registration, one needs a declaration of birth issued by a doctor as well as a request signed by both parents within two months of delivery (Abega 2007). In the case that the father does *not* recognize his child, his name will not appear on the birth certificate. Before 1981, however, mention would be made of "père inconnu,"

meaning "unknown father" (Calvès 2000). In the absence of a cooperative partner, or of a medical birth declaration, women can also obtain a birth certificate later in the child's life. In this case, procedures are more complicated and should pass through court—a process that costs 2,000 CFA francs, plus the bribes for the intermediaries and officials in charge. For villagers in Asung, such a belated registration often comes down to a total sum of 5,000 CFA francs (around 7.5 euros). Birth certificates are deemed important in the lives of Cameroonian citizens because they are required for a national identity card, school enrollment, and job applications. The daily newspaper *Mutation* once reported the problems that appear when primary school pupils want to take their final exams but are unable to show their birth certificates. The article mentioned a survey conducted in 2007 by the German NGO GTZ that showed that 36 percent of the ten thousand surveyed teenage mothers encountered difficulties with obtaining birth certificates. The problem seems to be biggest in the East and Extreme North Provinces (Gaïbaï 2009).

29. Although I present the possible etiological explanations here in terms of broader "categories" (discovered through the methods of free listing and pile sorting), I do not pretend to give an all-encompassing, coherent account of what turned out to be varied and contradicting descriptions. See also Pool (2003).

CHAPTER 5

1. I understand "distress" not only in physical terms but also, in line with Nichter (1981: 403), as "a broad range of feeling states including vulnerability, apprehension, inadequacy, dissatisfaction, suppressed anger and other anxiety states which might otherwise take the form of an untenable social conflict or rebellion." I agree with Nichter that idioms expressing these feelings "are culturally constituted in the sense that they initiate particular types of interaction and are associated with culturally pervasive values, norms, generative themes, and health concerns" (379). This chapter will explore such idioms and the underlying meanings and implications for particular types of interaction in the Gbigbil village of Asung.

2. Seying ining is a women's association initiated by Plan International, the only international NGO present in Asung. In 2009, it had twenty-eight members (twenty-two women and six men). The association has multiple goals: to provide women with agricultural tools and knowledge so as to promote their economic independence; to encourage cooperation by creating female "working groups" on a communal cassava field and "support groups" in case of misfortune; to provide support for, and create awareness of, hospital

services and medical interventions, especially in the domain of mother and child health; and to take care of orphans. Despite its presence and impetus for activities in the village, Plan International is surrounded by suspicion and ambivalence in Asung. Many villagers complain of the corruption that must be present at higher levels since they "never receive anything." Similar assumptions extend to mama Rosie and other representatives, who are suspected of receiving money for their activities in the village—which, in fact, they do not.

3.   An *agent de santé* (health agent) or *délégué de santé* (health delegate) is a community member who is part of the community's *committee de santé* (COSA; health committee), which also has a president, a secretary, and a treasurer. Health committees are supposed to collaborate closely with local health centers. They were installed after the Cameroonian government revised the primary health care approach in 1987 and proposed a decentralization of decision-making power into peripheral hands. The particular role of agents de santé like mama Rosie is to create health awareness among their fellow villagers, to encourage hospital visits for routine check-ups or vaccinations, to distribute health-related messages and products (such as mosquito nets), and to gather health statistics (especially about mother and child health). Agents de santé have been trained and should ideally receive a small remuneration for their activities. In practice, however, collaboration and communication with the health center is often lacking, and payment postponed or completely absent.

4.   As mentioned in Chapter 3, Gbigbil funeral ceremonies consist of quasi-humorous ritual interactions (*saŋba*) between in-married wives and native daughters of Asung. They offers in-married wives like mama Rosie an opportunity to denounce the ambiguities of their own status as outsiders, and to ridicule their families-in-law (especially mothers-in-law) in ways that are otherwise not accepted.

5.   This training in housekeeping chores (cooking, cleaning, sewing) for young women was part of the Catholic mission in Diang, some twenty kilometers from mama Rosie's natal village.

6.   It remains unclear whether this particular confession really took place. Different ethnographic sources have noted, however, that witchcraft confessions are increasingly present in the region. While many of these are forcefully or indirectly uttered in court, others are willfully (though privately) conceded in order to enhance a process of healing; one cannot be cured as long as one has not confessed past deeds and hidden powers. Such confessions are not always negatively evaluated, since they might prevent worse things from happening (Fisiy and Geschiere 1990; Geschiere 1997b; Geschiere and Fisiy 1994).

7. Formal marriage acts can be signed for monogamous or polygynous unions. This case obviously concerns a formal polygynous marriage.

8. According to traditions, daughters-in-law need to offer the first products of their fields to their parents-in-law. This *tjəŋ*, as it is called, might be fresh corn-cobs or corn-based preparations such as couscous. The in-laws are supposed to give a symbolic amount of money in return, whereupon the daughter-in-law is allowed to consume her own production for the rest of the year. If *tjəŋ* obligations are not respected, harvests might get spoiled. In practice, however, many women do neglect their *tjəŋ* duties or give it to another person if relations with the in-laws are not good.

9. This center is part of the Provincial Delegation of the Ministry of Women's Empowerment and Family. It aims to offer (1) training for women's economic, social, and cultural empowerment; (2) education on responsible parenthood and on mother and child health; (3) support for women's entrepreneurship; and (4) improvement of the living and working conditions of urban and rural women. The specific center in Bertoua that Laura mentions provides trainings for women in sewing, informatics, nursery care, and cooking; reproductive health services such as prenatal consultations, routine vaccinations, HIV/AIDS screening, and educational talks about hygiene, pregnancy, and contraception; informative sessions about legal family affairs (such as marriage and birth certificates or inheritance laws); and funding for (thirty-nine) initiatives and projects aimed at women's empowerment.

10. Pope John Paul II visited Cameroon on August 10–14, 1985, and September 14–16, 1995. Pope Benedict XVI followed him on March 16–19, 2009. In 1985, Pope John Paul II held a service at Bamenda Airport in which he referred to "God's plan for marriage and the family 'from the beginning.'" In covert terms, he talked about abortion when he condemned the increasing presence of a "powerful anti-life mentality" and argued human life to be "a splendid gift of God's goodness" that should never be harmed (*w2.vatican.va/content/john-paul-ii/en/homilies/1985/documents/hf_jp-ii_hom_19850812_famiglie-bamenda.html*). It is probably this discourse that inspired Laura—albeit her interpretation had turned the pope's words into a curse.

11. Quinine is a bitter alkaloid with fever-reducing, antimalarial, analgesic, and anti-inflammatory properties, which is believed to function as an abortifacient if taken in large quantities. *Kangwa* is a "traditional salt" (a condiment) that is often used in local medicinal compositions. *Cytotec* is a drug containing misoprostol, which causes uterine contractions and dilation of the cervix. It is used to instigate problematic spontaneous pregnancy interruptions, to provoke early abortions, or to induce labor.

12. Such feminists have attacked earlier theories that, from the mid-1970s onward, speculated about women's innate role as mothers. Examples of those essentialist treatises are Klaus and Kennel's (1976) work on "maternal bonding" and Ruddick's (1980) idea of "maternal thinking." The feminist theoretical framework that, in reaction, took gender subordination (and the psychological processes it involves—see Chodorow [1978] and Gilligan [1982]) as its starting point and posited women as victims came to be called "dominance feminism." Within this framework, patriarchy is seen as a total system of "gender oppression" or as "male domination/female subordination." Such a perspective differs from the anthropological one, which locates patriarchy within the domestic realm and family life. Inhorn (1996: 3–4) merges these two approaches into one overarching definition, stating that "patriarchy is characterized by relations of power and authority of males over females, which are 1) learned through gender socialization within the family, where males wield power through the socially defined institution of fatherhood; 2) manifested in both inter- and intragender interactions within the family and in other interpersonal milieus; 3) legitimized through deeply engrained, pervasive ideologies of inherent male superiority; and 4) institutionalized on many societal levels (legal, political, economic, educational, religious, and so on)." The author further contends that pronatalism is deeply engrained in patriarchy. Whenever I talk about patriarchy in this chapter, I take this all-encompassing definition as a starting point.

13. Gerrits (2002) presents an overview of anthropological literature in which this line of thinking is confirmed. She states how the lives of infertile women in patrilineal African communities have generally been depicted "as marked by suffering and exclusion" (234). Gerrits draws a different conclusion based on fieldwork among a matrilineal community in Mozambique. While her attempt to move away from a discourse of suffering around infertility is laudable, the fact that she attributes women's different experiences to the matrilineal system leaves the assumptions related to patriarchy unquestioned.

14. See J. Fischer (2003), Hanigsberg (1995), Hewson (2001), Kim (1999), Meyers (2001), Petchesky (1980), and Thomson (1971).

15. Of course, this broad generalization does not do justice to some excellent and detailed studies that have described the complex power intricacies in both abortion cases and infertility experiences all over the world. See, for instance, Feldman-Savelsberg (1999), Gerrits (2016), Ginsburg (1998), Inhorn (1996, 2012), Monach (1993), Olarte Sierra (2010), Rapp (2000), and Whittaker (2002, 2004).

16. See Connell (1997), Inhorn (1996), Kandiyoti (1988), Lock and Kaufert (1997), and Mahoney (1994). Some feminists have proposed to work with

the concept of *relational autonomy* (Mackenzie and Stoljar 2000; Nguyen 2011; Pollack 2000; Schneider 1993). In highlighting the social embedded-ness of agency, the concept explores "the space between women's victimiza-tion and oppression and women's active responses to these conditions, and in so doing helps to dislodge the victim/agent dichotomy" (Pollack 2000: 84).

17. Inherent to this development thinking is a discourse of individual self-improvement and self-actualization. This individualistic notion of empower-ment, as well as the linearity that underlies it, has been criticized by Cornwall (2007a) and by feminists who see autonomy as a *relational* affair (see the previous note).

18. In his review of infertility studies in Cameroon, Lantum (1976) has drawn attention to the absence of (demographic and other) studies on abortions in the face of a whole body of literature on infertility. The contribution of abortions to the problem of infertility and low fertility therefore remains unknown. See also the work of Cates et al. (1985), David and Voas (1981), Ericksen and Brunette (1996), Frank (1983), Larsen (1995), Nasah (1978), Retel-Laurentin (1974), and Romaniuk (1961, 1968) on infertility in Cameroon.

19. In this diary excerpt (nos. 703–5), Father Willem de Jong explicitly focused his attention on marriage traditions and family life in Cameroon. He described the four issues in detail and situated them within relevant social and historical contexts. Through this contextualization, he argued for a more comprehensive understanding of, and flexible adaptation to, encoun-tered realities in the field. This excerpt was retrieved at the archives of the Congregatio Sancti Spiritus in Gemert, the Netherlands, in August 2007.

20. Sixa (allegedly a derivative of the English word "sister") was promoted as a school where young women would receive proper education in Christian dogma as well as in household and conjugal affairs before their baptism and marriage in church. Many women of various ages and backgrounds gathered in the sixa for different periods of time, depending on their level of education and conduct (Criaud 1990; Vincent 2001). "Free" daughters were sent by their parents or forced by missionaries to participate. Other young women were sent by their Christian fiancés who anticipated a religious marriage immediately after the training. Further, as a pathway toward a monogamous Christian marriage, sixa also appealed to those who found themselves in polygynous unions or in otherwise badly perceived marriages. They joined the sixa to get rest and enjoy the harmony between "sisters" rather than to become a Christian wife.

21. This ministry was officially installed through decree no. 2005–088 of March 29, 2005. It united the former Ministry of Social Affairs (MINAS, created

in 1975) and the Ministry of Women's Conditions (MINCOF, created in 1984), which temporarily merged into the Ministry of Social Affairs and Women's Conditions (MINASCOF) between 1988 and 1997. The ministry is currently in charge of: the elaboration and implementation of measures relating to Cameroonian women's rights in society; the elimination of all forms of discrimination against women; the increase in chances for equality in political, economic, social and cultural domains; and the implementation of the national policy on families.

22. Several ethnographic sources have made a similar point by showing the possibility for female revolt in the patriarchal order. See, for instance, Abega (2007), Ardener (1973), Barbier (1985), Copet-Rougier (1985), Geschiere (1985), Laburthe-Tolra (1981), and Nkwi (1985).

23. Remarkably, while expressions of suffering are abundant, utterances of particular emotional states are almost absent in Gbigbil women's narratives. As is described by Nichter (1981) for Indian women as well, it seems that somatic complaints or symbolic idioms of distress take precedence over concrete discussions about affects and sentiments, whether related to pregnancy interruptions or other experiences. My in-depth analysis of women's complaints of suffering within particular social situations will, however, partly reveal the emotional states and tensions that underlie these idioms of distress.

24. A similar interpretation of suffering as strength surrounds birthing stories. My informants repeatedly stressed that only *women* could endure labor pains and other forms of reproductive suffering. Their idea that men would "not be able to endure these agonies" strengthens the notion of a shared female power.

25. Tellingly, a focus group discussion on agency and suffering was filled with women's constant referrals to themselves as the ones who suffered most—which, apart from creating the atmosphere of mutual understanding that I had hoped for, led to a sort of contest between women impressing each other by their display of personal misery. The acknowledgment of suffering as a marker of good womanhood formed not only a source of solidarity, but also a source of competition and distinction, between women.

26. A report in the archives of the Congregatio Sancti Spiritus in Gemert, the Netherlands, notes that, "Due to the underpopulation—109,000 km² for 600,000 inhabitants—in the East Province of Cameroon, the accent has been laid on procreation. Children should be born, whether in a normal union or outside of marriage."

27. Similar attitudes have been found elsewhere in and outside of Cameroon. See Bleek (1976), Copet-Rougier (1985), Feldman-Savelsberg (1999), Inhorn (1994, 1996), Kielmann (1998), Leonard (2002), Nahar (2007), Njikam Savage (1992), and Sundby et al. (1998).

28. Tellingly, the theft of one of my own freshly washed panties caused serious concerns regarding the implications it could have for my future fertility if the thief would turn out to be a witch.

29. Artificial donor insemination was introduced in 1985 in the department of Obstetrics and Gynecology of the University Hospital Center (UHC) in Yaoundé, and subsequently at the Central Maternity in the same city. While both institutions offered services up to 1989, nowadays infertility treatment can be obtained only at the Central Maternity. It is, however, largely inaccessible—geographically, financially, and socioculturally—to most Cameroonians. Local cultural frameworks that deny the existence of male infertility form the most important sociocultural barrier to artificial donor insemination (Feldman-Savelsberg 2002; Njikam Savage 1992).

30. See de Rosny (1974), de Thé (1970), Johnson et al. (1990), Mallart Guimera (1981), Richards (2002), and van Beek (1994).

31. Stories about men's "true love" for childless women are quite common in the village. One day, I witnessed an old man dancing and singing on the street. People explained to me that he was singing about his first wife who had not been able to conceive and had been chased by her family-in-law. The man had married a second, fertile wife but still regretted the departure of the first one; "they had chased away his heart." Inhorn (1996: 9) also notes that, even in a strict "classical" patriarchal society like Egypt, infertility might actually strengthen the "connectivity" between a husband and his infertile wife, expressed in terms of intense love, involvement, and commitment.

32. Fosterage practices are widespread in Cameroon and other West African countries. See the work of Alber (2003), Carsten (2004), Einarsdóttir (2006), Eloundou-Enyegue and Stokes (2009), Goody (1984), Notermans (2003, 2008), and Verhoef (2005).

33. This is well above the estimated Cameroonian fosterage rate of 25 percent (Eloundou-Enyegue and Stokes 2009: 282), the exact calculation of which is however not clarified. It might mean that 25 percent of the women are fostering children—in which case the rate is comparable to the 49 percent found in my survey. But it might also mean that 25 percent of all children are fostered.

34. More precisely, there is one law in the Code of Canon Law that refers specifically to abortion. This is canon 1398, which states, "A person who procures a completed abortion incurs a *latae sententiae* [automatic] excommunication" (Barzelatto 2004). The church distinguishes between "direct" and "indirect" abortion. Indirect abortion is defined as the killing of a fetus in the course of another medical intervention necessary to save a woman's life. Because such an intervention is not aimed at the destruction of the fetus, it is not morally

condemned. The church does condemn direct abortion, even if procured to save a woman's life. This type of abortion is permitted in Cameroonian law and approved by most people in Asung.

35. An example is the prochoice organization Catholics for Choice, based in Washington, DC. It was founded in 1973 "to serve as a voice for Catholics who believe that the Catholic tradition supports a woman's moral and legal right to follow her conscience in matters of sexuality and reproductive health." The organization aims to ensure that all people have access to safe and affordable reproductive health care services.

36. They protested against article 14 on Health and Reproductive Rights, which proposes to "protect the reproductive rights of women by authorizing medical abortion in cases of sexual assault, rape, incest, and where the continued pregnancy endangers the mental and physical health of the mother or the life of the mother or the fetus" (African Union 2003: 16). The "national committee of human rights and liberties" then reacted to this situation by organizing an "explicatory conference" on the consequences of the Maputo protocol for Cameroon. The few individual efforts and awareness-raising campaigns of NGOs like the Association de Lutte contre les Violences faites aux Femmes (ALVF) that happened afterward have had little influence at national and legal levels.

37. Given the formal disapproval surrounding the topic, as well as my own outsider status and probable association with formal institutions, the real incidence of abortions is likely to be even higher. See also the work of Haws et al. (2010).

38. Similar motivations and abortion methods have been found in other studies in Cameroon and elsewhere. See Abega (2007), Bleek (1976, 1981), Calvès (2002, 2009), CEPED (2000), Feldman-Savelsberg, Schuster, and Ndonko (2008), Guttmacher Institute (2003), Henshaw et al. (1999), Johnson-Hanks (2002a), Koster (2003), Nyobia (2006), Renne (1996, 2006), and Schuster (2005).

39. This tactical deployment of the patriarchal discourse might have negative repercussions for men. Feminist assumptions that patriarchal norms are always automatically directed against women should thus be more nuanced and considered from the men's perspective as well.

40. This fear is not unwarranted: the most recent statistics from the Cameroonian Demographic and Health Survey (DHS) in 2011 show an alarming maternal mortality rate of 782 per 100,000 live births, of which a considerable part is probably caused by abortion-related complications. Koster (2010), Renne (2006), and Schuster (2010) also mention the direct relation between abortions and infertility or death in the region.

CONCLUSION

1. Especially in the East Province, men and women alike are described as being in a permanent quest for children—for both economic and ideological reasons (Wakam 1994). The considerable sexual liberty granted to girls and women in the East of Cameroon is further seen as leading to abundant childbearing in and out of wedlock and has been contrasted with, for example, the Bamiléké people in the West of Cameroon, who are seen as much more calculating regarding both economic and reproductive matters (Feldman-Savelsberg 1999; Yana 1995).

2. It should be noted that fertility interruptions can be the *cause* of this flow of decisions (especially when the mishap happens unexpectedly and seems to endanger previous pathways or projects), or their *result* (especially when the pregnancy is purposefully interrupted because it seems to endanger [possible] pathways or projects). Nevertheless, I argue that these questions influence women's reproductive navigation in the broader conjunctures around *any* pregnancy interruption, whether spontaneous or induced.

3. In his conceptualization of coincidence, the sociologist Howard Becker (1994) also mentions the notion of intercontingency. Though he does not define the concept, it becomes clear that what he means is the interdependency between individual actions and choices on the one hand, and the actions and choices that other persons make (or have been making) as a result of contingencies in *their* lives, on the other.

4. Guyer's broader argument posits that the focus on originality and self-realization resulted in, and was the result of, the societal production of "*multiplicity* amongst *singular* people who were each at their own frontier of experience" (1996: 2, emphasis in original). Personal specializations within a particular domain of knowledge or expertise did not only induce and sustain processes of distinction and diversification at the micro level but also led to interpersonal complementarity that ensured the success of the larger social order.

5. These idioms carry different connotations than witchcraft stories in, for instance, the western part of Cameroon, where power has long been centralized and different dynamics are at play (see Fisiy and Geschiere 1993).

6. Surprisingly, in the rest of the article from which this quote is taken, Lock reviews in particular studies that have interpreted bodies in terms of their sociality rather than their materiality (1993a). Other scholars (see, for instance, Kirmayer 1992; Lyon 1997) have criticized this trend in anthropology to either ignore or symbolize the body and argue for a recognition of its material aspects as well.

Bibliography

Abega, S. C. (2007). Les *violences sexuelles et l'état au Cameroun*. Paris: Karthala.

Aboubakar, A. (2008). *Perceptions et pratiques des soins obstétricaux traditionnels chez les Pèrè de Gadjiwan (Prince de l'Adamaoua, Cameroun)*. Yaoundé: Université de Yaoundé I.

Adetunji, J. A. (1996). "Preserving the Pot and Water: A Traditional Concept of Reproductive Health in a Yoruba Community, Nigeria." *Social Science and Medicine, 43*(11), 1561–76.

African Union. (2003). *Protocol to the African Charter on Human and Peoples' Rights on the Rights of Women in Africa*. Maputo: African Union.

Ako, S., Fokoua, S., Sinou, M. T., and Leke, R. (2003). "Reproductive Health in Cameroon." [Electronic version.] Retrieved March 3, 2007, from *www.gfmer.ch/ Endo/Reprod_health/Cameroon/Net_Reproduction_Cameroun.htm*.

Akuri, J., Weinger, S., and Barton, B. (2009). "When Personal Dreams Derail, Rural Cameroonian Women Aspire for Their Children." *Journal of International Women's Studies, 11*(2), 142–56.

Alber, E. (2003). "Denying Biological Parenthood: Fosterage in Northern Benin." *Ethnos, 68*(4), 487–506.

Allen, D. R. (2002). *Managing Motherhood, Managing Risk: Fertility and Danger in West Central Tanzania*. Ann Arbor: University of Michigan Press.

Appadurai, A. (2004). "The Capacity to Aspire: Culture and the Terms of Recognition." In V. Rao and M. Walton (Eds.), *Culture and Public Action: A Cross-Disciplinary Dialogue on Development Policy* (pp. 59–84). Palo Alto, CA: Stanford University Press.

Ardener, S. G. (1973). Sexual Insult and Female Militancy. *Man, 8*(3), 422–40.

Asowa-Omorodion, F. I. (1997). "Women's Perceptions of the Complications of Pregnancy and Childbirth in Two Esan Communities, Edo State, Nigeria." *Social Science and Medicine, 44*(12), 1817–24.

Atangana, S. (1998). "Aperçu historique de la mise en oeuvre des soins de santé primaires au Cameroun." In Ministère de la Santé Publique Cameroun (Ed.),

La mise en oeuvre de la réorientation des soins de santé primaires au Cameroun. Yaoundé: Ministère de la Santé Publique.

Bahanag, A. M. B. (2003). *Politiques démographiques, traditions natalistes et développement durable au Cameroun.* Yaoundé: Université de Yaoundé I.

Balla, C. (1991). *Parole et pouvoir chez les Beti (Cameroun Central): Approche ethnolinguistique.* Yaoundé: Université de Yaoundé I.

Barbier, J.-C. (1985). *Femmes du Cameroun: Mères pacifiques, femmes rebelles.* Paris: Karthala.

Barzelatto, J. (2004). *Catholics on Abortion.* Washington, DC: Catholics for a Free Choice.

Basu, A. M. (2002). "Why Does Education Lead to Lower Fertility? A Critical Review of Some of the Possibilities." *World Development, 30*(10), 1779–90.

Bauvineau, L. (2004). *Histoire de l'église Catholique dans l'Est du Cameroun.* Czestochowa: Educator.

Becker, G. (1994). "Metaphors in Disrupted Lives: Infertility and Cultural Constructions of Continuity." *Medical Anthropology Quarterly, 8*(4), 383–410.

———. (2000). *The Elusive Embryo: How Women and Men Approach New Reproductive Technologies.* Berkeley: University of California Press.

Becker, H. S. (1994). "'Foi por Acaso': Conceptualizing Coincidence." *Sociological Quarterly, 35*(2), 183–94.

Beninguissé, G. (2003). *Entre tradition et modernité: Fondements sociaux de la prise en charge de la grossesse et de l'accouchement au Cameroun.* Louvain-la-Neuve: Bruylant-Academia.

———. (2010). "Les politiques de santé de la reproduction en Afrique depuis la conférence du Caire: Quelles implications pour la régulation de la fécondité?" In R. Fassassi, K. Vignikin, and P. Vimard (Eds.), *La régulation de la fécondité en Afrique: Transformations et différenciations au tournant du XXIe siècle* (pp. 23–38). Louvain-la-Neuve: Academia-Bruylant.

Bhattacharya, S., Prescott, G. J., Black, M., and Shetty, A. (2010). "Recurrence Risk of Stillbirth in a Second Pregnancy." *BJOG: An International Journal of Obstetrics and Gynaecology, 117*(10), 1243–47.

Biehl, J. G., Good, B., and Kleinman, A. (2007). *Subjectivity: Ethnographic Investigations.* Berkeley: University of California Press.

Billard, P. (1961). *La circulation dans le Sud Cameroun.* Lyon: Impression des Beaux-Arts.

Bledsoe, C. (2002). *Contingent Lives: Fertility, Time, and Aging in West Africa.* Chicago: University of Chicago Press.

Bledsoe, C., Banja, F., and Hill, A. G. (1998). "Reproductive Mishaps and Western Contraception: An African Challenge to Fertility Theory." *Population and Development Review, 24*(1), 15–58.

Bledsoe, C., Casterline, J. B., Johnson-Kuhn, J. A., and Haaga, J. G. (1999). *Critical Perspectives on Schooling and Fertility in the Developing World.* Washington, DC: National Academy Press.

Bledsoe, C., and Cohen, B. (1993). *Social Dynamics of Adolescent Fertility in Sub-Saharan Africa.* Washington, DC: National Academy Press.

Bledsoe, C., and Scherrer, R. F. (2007). "The Dialectics of Disruption: Paradoxes of Nature and Professionalism in Contemporary American Childbearing." In M. C. Inhorn (Ed.), *Reproductive Disruptions: Gender, Technology, and Biopolitics in the New Millennium* (pp. 47–78). New York: Berghahn Books.

Bleek, W. (1976). *Sexual Relationships and Birthcontrol in Ghana: A Case Study of a Rural Town.* Amsterdam: Antropologisch Sociologisch Centrum.

———. (1981). "Avoiding Shame: The Ethical Context of Abortion in Ghana." *Anthropological Quarterly, 54*(4), 203–9.

Boddy, J. (1989). *Wombs and Alien Spirits: Women, Men, and the Zar Cult in Northern Sudan.* Madison: University of Wisconsin Press.

Boerma, J. T., and Mgalla, Z. (2001). *Women and Infertility in Sub-Saharan Africa: A Multi-disciplinary Perspective.* Amsterdam: Royal Tropical Institute Press.

Bonnet, D. (1988). *Corps biologique, corps social: Procréation et maladies de l'enfant en pays mossi, Burkina Faso.* Paris: ORSTOM.

Boulenger, D., Barten, F., and Criel, B. (2014). "Contracting between Faith-Based Health Care Organizations and the Public Sector in Africa." *Review of Faith and International Affairs, 12*(1), 21–29.

Bourdieu, P. (1977). *Outline of a Theory of Practice.* Cambridge: Cambridge University Press.

———. (1989). "Social Space and Symbolic Power." *Sociological Theory, 7*(1), 14–25.

Braudel, F. (1980). *On History.* Chicago: University of Chicago Press.

Brigham, S. A., Conlon, C., and Farquharson, R. G. (1999). "A Longitudinal Study of Pregnancy Outcome Following Idiopathic Recurrent Miscarriage." *Human Reproduction, 14,* 2868–71.

Bury, M. (1982). "Chronic Illness as Biographical Disruption." *Sociology of Health and Illness, 4*(2), 167–82.

Calvès, A. E. (1999). "Marginalization of African Single Mothers in the Marriage Market: Evidence from Cameroon." *Population Studies, 53*(3), 291–301.

———. (2000). "Premarital Childbearing in Urban Cameroon: Paternal Recognition, Child Care and Financial Support." *Journal of Comparative Family Studies, 31*(4), 443–61.

———. (2002). "Abortion Risk and Decisionmaking among Young People in Urban Cameroon." *Studies in Family Planning, 33*(3), 249–60.

———. (2009). "Décision d'avorter et déterminants des avortements clandestins chez les jeunes de Yaoundé." In C. Gourbin (Ed.), *Santé de la reproduction au Nord et au Sud: De la connaissance à l'action* (pp. 439–56). Louvain-la-Neuve: Les Presses Universitaires de Louvain.

Calvès, A. E., and Meekers, D. (1999). "The Advantages of Having Many Children for Women in Formal and Informal Unions in Cameroon." *Journal of Comparative Family Studies, 30*(4), 617–39.

Carsten, J. (2000). *Cultures of Relatedness: New Approaches to the Study of Kinship.* Cambridge: Cambridge University Press.

———. (2004). *After Kinship.* Cambridge: Cambridge University Press.

Casper, M. J. (1998). *The Making of the Unborn Patient: A Social Anatomy of Fetal Surgery.* New Brunswick, NJ: Rutgers University Press.

Cates, W., Farley, T. M. M., and Rowe, P. J. (1985). "Worldwide Patterns of Infertility: Is Africa Different?" *Lancet, 14*, 596–98.

Cecil, R. (1996). *The Anthropology of Pregnancy Loss: Comparative Studies in Miscarriage, Stillbirth, and Neonatal Death.* Oxford: Berg.

CEPED (Centre Population et Développement) (2000). "Loi sur l'avortement." *La chronique du Ceped, 37*, 1–8.

Chapman, R. R. (2003). "Endangering Safe Motherhood in Mozambique: Prenatal Care as Pregnancy Risk." *Social Science and Medicine, 57*(2), 355–74.

———. (2010). *Family Secrets: Risking Reproduction in Central Mozambique.* Nashville, TN: Vanderbilt University Press.

Chodorow, N. (1978). *The Reproduction of Mothering.* Berkeley: University of California Press.

Corbett, M. R., and Turner, K. L. (2003). "Essential Elements of Postabortion Care: Origins, Evolution and Future Directions." *International Family Planning Perspectives, 29*, 106–11.

Clifford, K., Rai, R., and Regan, L. (1997). "Future Pregnancy Outcome in Unexplained Recurrent First Trimester Miscarriage." *Human Reproduction, 12*, 387–89.

Cole, J. (2010). *Sex and Salvation: Imagining the Future in Madagaskar.* Chicago: University of Chicago Press.

Cole, J., and Durham, D. L. (2008). *Figuring the Future: Globalization and the Temporalities of Children and Youth*. Santa Fe, NM: School for Advanced Research Press.

Commission Nationale de la Population Cameroun. (1993). *National Population Policy Declaration*. Yaoundé: Commission Nationale de la Population Cameroun.

Connell, P. (1997). "Understanding Victimization and Agency: Considerations of Race, Class and Gender." *Political and Legal Anthropology Review, 20*(2), 115–43.

Copet-Rougier, E. (1985). "Controle masculin, exclusivité féminine dans une société patrilinéaire." In J.-C. Barbier (Ed.), *Femmes du Cameroun: Mères pacifiques, femmes rebelles* (pp. 153–80). Paris: Karthala.

———. (1987). "Du clan à la chefferie dans l'Est du Cameroun." *Africa, 57*, 345–63.

———. (1998). "Political-Economic History of the Upper-Sangha." *Forestry and Environmental Studies Bulletin, 102*, 51–71.

Cornwall, A. (2007a). "Of Choice, Chance and Contingency: 'Career Strategies' and Tactics for Survival among Yoruba Women Traders." *Social Anthropology, 15*(1), 27–46.

———. (2007b). "Taking Chances, Making Choices: The Tactical Dimensions of 'Reproductive Strategies' in Southwestern Nigeria." *Medical Anthropology, 26*(3), 229–54.

Criaud, J. (1990). *La geste des Spiritains: Histoire de l'Église au Cameroun*. Yaoundé: Publications du centenaire.

Csordas, T. J. (1990). "Embodiment as a Paradigm for Anthropology." *Ethos, 18*(1), 5–47.

———. (1994). *Embodiment and Experience: The Existential Ground of Culture and Self*. Cambridge: Cambridge University Press.

David, N., and Voas, D. (1981). "Societal Causes of Infertility and Population Decline among the Settled Fulani of North Cameroon." *Man, 16*(4), 644–64.

de Bruyn, M. (2003). "Safe Abortion for HIV-Positive Women with Unwanted Pregnancy: A Reproductive Right." *Reproductive Health Matters, 11*(22), 152–61.

de Certeau, M. (1984). *The Practice of Everyday Life*. Berkeley: University of California Press.

de Lesdain, S. B. (1998). "Sexualité et procréation chez les Mvae (Cameroun)." *Autrepart, 7*, 139–52.

Delpech, B. (1985). "Femmes éton devant les tribunaux coutumiers." In J.-C. Barbier (Ed.), *Femmes du Cameroun: Meres pacifiques, femmes rebelles* (pp. 327–40). Paris: Karthala.

Denzin, N. K. (2001). *Interpretive Interactionism*. London: Sage.

de Rosny, É. (1974). *Ndimsi: Ceux qui soignent dans la nuit.* Yaoundé: Editions CLE.

de Thé, M. P. (1970). *Des sociétés secrètes aux associations modernes: La femme dans la dynamique de la société Beti, 1887–1966.* Paris: Ecole Pratique des Hautes Études.

Devisch, R. (1993). *Weaving the Threads of Life: The Khita Gyn-Eco-Logical Healing Cult among the Yaka.* Chicago: University of Chicago Press.

DHS. (2011). *Demographic and Health Survey Cameroon.* Calverton: ICF International.

Dimmock, F., Olivier, J., and Wodon, Q. (2012). "Half a Century Young: The Christian Health Associations in Africa." In J. Olivier and Q. Wodon (Eds.), *The Role of Faith-Inspired Health Care Providers in Sub-Saharan Africa and Public-Private Partnerships.* Washington, DC: World Bank.

Douglas, M. (1966). *Purity and Danger: An Analysis of Concept of Pollution and Taboo.* London: Routledge.

Downe, S., and Dykes, F. (2009). "Counting Time in Pregnancy and Labour." In C. McCourt (Ed.), *Childbirth, Midwifery and Concepts of Time* (pp. 61–83). New York: Berghahn Books.

Duden, B. (1993). *Disembodying Women: Perspectives on Pregnancy and the Unborn.* Cambridge, MA: Harvard University Press.

Dugast, I. (1949). *Inventaire Ethnique du Sud-Cameroun.* Douala: Institut français d'Afrique noire.

Dunkle, K. L., Jewkes, R., Nduna, M., Jama, N., Levin, J., Sikweyiya, Y., et al. (2007). "Transactional Sex with Casual and Main Partners among Young South African Men in the Rural Eastern Cape: Prevalence, Predictors, and Associations with Gender-Based Violence." *Social Science and Medicine, 65*(6), 1235–48.

Earle, S. (2004). "'Planned' and 'Unplanned' Pregnancy: Deconstructing Experiences of Conception." *Human Fertility, 17*(1), 39–42.

Earle, S., Foley, P., Komaromy, C., and Lloyd, C. (2008). "Conceptualizing Reproductive Loss: A Social Sciences Perspective." *Human Fertility, 11*(4), 259–62.

Earle, S., and Letherby, G. (2002). "Whose Choice Is It Anyway? Decision Making, Control and Conception." *Human Fertility, 5*(2), 39–41.

———. (2007). "Conceiving Time? Women Who Do or Do Not Conceive." *Sociology of Health and Illness, 29*(2), 233–50.

Einarsdóttir, J. (2000). *"Tired of Weeping": Child Death and Mourning among Papel Mothers in Guinea-Bissau.* Stockholm: Almqvist and Wiksell.

———. (2006). "Relocation of Children: Fosterage and Child Death in Biombo, Guinea-Bissau." In C. Christiansen, M. Utas, and H. E. Vigh (Eds.), *Navigating Youth, Generating Adulthood: Social Becoming in an African Context* (pp. 154–83). Uppsala: Nordiska Afrikainstitutet.

———. (2009). "Emotional Experts: Parents' Views on End-of-Life Decisions for Preterm Infants in Iceland." *Medical Anthropology Quarterly, 23*(1), 34–50.

Eloundou-Enyegue, P. M. (2004). "Pregnancy-Related Dropouts and Gender Inequality in Education: A Life-Table Approach and Application to Cameroon." *Demography, 41*(3), 509–28.

Eloundou-Enyegue, P. M., Ngoube, M., Okene, R., Onguene, V., Bahoken, S., Tamukong, T., et al. (2004). "Access to Schooling and Employment in Cameroon: New Inequalities and Opportunities." Strategies and Analysis for Growth and Access (SAGA). Working Paper, Cornell and Clark-Atlanta Universities, Ithaca, New York.

Eloundou-Enyegue, P. M., and Stokes, C. S. (2009). "Will Economic Crises in Africa Weaken Rural-Urban Ties? Insights from Child Fosterage Trends in Cameroon." *Rural Sociology, 67*(2), 278–98.

Ericksen, K., and Brunette, T. (1996). "Patterns and Predictors of Infertility among African Women: A Cross-National Survey of Twenty-Seven Nations." *Social Science and Medicine, 42*(2), 209–20.

Erny, P. (1988). *Les premiers pas dans la vie de l'enfant d'Afrique Noire: Naissance et première enfance.* Paris: L'Harmattan.

Erviti, J., Castro, R., and Collado, A. (2004). "Strategies Used by Low-Income Mexican Women to Deal with Miscarriage and Spontaneous Abortion." *Qualitative Health Research, 14*(8), 1058–76.

Eschlimann, J. P. (1982). *Naître sur la terre Africaine.* Abidjan: Inades.

Eto, G. S. (2005). *Genre et recours thérapeutique au Cameroun.* Yaoundé: IFORD.

Evina Mbo, F. I. (2005). *Les facteurs explicatifs du multipartenariat sexuel au Cameroun.* Yaoundé: IFORD.

Feldman-Savelsberg, P. (1996). "Cooking Inside: Kinship and Gender in Bangangté Idioms of Marriage and Procreation." In M. J. Maynes (Ed.), *Gender, Kinship, Power: A Comparative and Interdisciplinary History* (pp. 176–97). New York: Routledge.

———. (1999). *Plundered Kitchens, Empty Wombs: Threatened Reproduction and Identity in the Cameroon Grassfields.* Ann Arbor: University of Michigan Press.

———. (2002). "Is Infertility an Unrecognized Public Health and Population Problem?" In M. C. Inhorn and F. v. Balen (Eds.), *Infertility around the Globe: New Thinking on Childlessness, Gender, and Reproductive Technologies* (pp. 215–32). Berkeley: University of California Press.

Feldman-Savelsberg, P., Ndonko, F., and Yang, S. (2006). "The Social Management of Fetal and Infant Death: Dual Disruptions to Reproductive Lives and Discourses." *Curare, 29*(1), 17–26.

Feldman-Savelsberg, P., Schuster, S., and Ndonko, F. (2008). "Common but Never Routine: A Differentiated View of Illegal Abortion in Cameroon." Paper presented at Reproductive Health Challenges: Multidisciplinary Approaches to Enhance Global Equity. Granvolden, Norway. August 27–29, 2008.

Fischer, J. M. (2003). "Abortion, Autonomy, and Control over One's Body." *Social Philosophy and Policy, 20*(2), 286–306.

Fischer, W., and Goblirsch, M. (2007). "Biographical Structuring: Narrating and Reconstructing the Self in Research and Professional Practice." In M. G. W. Bamberg (Ed.), *Narrative: State of the Art* (pp. 37–46). Amsterdam: John Benjamins.

Fischer-Rosenthal, W. (2000). "Biographical Work and Biographical Structuring in Present-Day Societies." In P. Chamberlayne, J. Bornat, and T. Wengraf (Eds.), *The Turn to Biographical Methods in Social Science: Comparative Issues and Examples* (pp. 109–25). London: Routledge.

Fisiy, C. F., and Geschiere, P. (1990). "Judges and Witches; or, How Is the State to Deal with Witchcraft? Examples from Southeast Cameroon." *Cahiers d'Etudes Africaines, 30*(118), 135–56.

———. (1993). "Sorcellerie et accumulation, variations régionales." In P. Geschiere and P. Konings (Eds.), *Itinéraires d'accumulation au Cameroun* (pp. 99–129). Paris: Karthala.

Fouda, M. (2004). *Je parle Camerounais: Pour un renouveau francofaune.* Paris: Karthala.

Frank, O. (1983). "Infertility in Sub-Saharan Africa: Estimates and Implications." *Population and Development Review, 9*(1), 137–44.

Franklin, S., and McKinnon, S. (2000). "New Directions in Kinship Study: A Core Concept Revisited." *Current Anthropology, 41*(2), 275–79.

Fru, A. E. (2008). *Traditional Birth Attendants and Maternal Delivery in the Mbatu Community (North West Province, Cameroon).* Yaoundé: Université de Yaoundé I.

Gaïbaï, D. (2009). "Mayo-Danay: 7.000 enfants sans acte de naissance." *Mutations,* March 31.

Gammeltoft, T. (2003a). "Between 'Science' and 'Superstition': Moral Perceptions of Induced Abortion among Young Adults in Vietnam." *Culture, Medicine and Psychiatry, 26*(3), 313–38.

———. (2003b). "The Ritualisation of Abortion in Contemporary Vietnam." *Australian Journal of Anthropology, 14*(2), 129–43.

———. (2006). "'Beyond Being': Emergent Narratives of Suffering in Vietnam." *Royal Anthropological Institute, 12*(3), 589–605.

———. (2010). "Between Remembering and Forgetting: Maintaining Moral Motherhood after Late-Term Abortion." In A. Whittaker (Ed.), *Abortion in Asia: Local Dilemmas, Global Politics* (pp. 56–77). New York: Berghahn Books.

Garenne, M. (2004). "Age at Marriage and Modernisation in Sub-Saharan Africa." *Southern African Journal of Demography, 9*(2), 59–79.

Gerber-Epstein, P., Leichtentritt, R., and Benyamini, Y. (2009). "The Experience of Miscarriage in First Pregnancy: The Women's Voices." *Death Studies, 33*(1), 1–29.

Gerring, J. (2007). *Case Study Research: Principles and Practice.* Cambridge: Cambridge University Press.

Gerrits, G. J. E. (2002). "Infertility and Matrilineality." In M. C. Inhorn and F. Van Balen (Eds.), *Infertility around the Globe: New Thinking on Childlessness, Gender, and Reproductive Technologies* (pp. 233–46). Berkeley: University of California Press.

———. (2016). *Patient-Centered IVF: Bioethics and Care in a Dutch Clinic.* New York: Berghahn Books.

Geschiere, P. (1982). *Village Communities and the State: Changing Relations among the Maka of South-Eastern Cameroon since the Colonial Conquest.* London: Kegan Paul International.

———. (1985). "La visite des belles-mères chez les Maka: Une rébellion contre les hommes?" In J.-C. Barbier (Ed.), *Femmes du Cameroun: Mères pacifiques, femmes rebelles* (pp. 194–216). Paris: Karthala.

———. (1997a). "Kinship, Witchcraft and the Market." In R. R. Grinker and C. B. Steiner (Eds.), *Perspectives on Africa: A Reader in Culture, History, and Representation* (pp. 340–58). Oxford: Blackwell.

———. (1997b). *The Modernity of Witchcraft: Politics and the Occult in Postcolonial Africa.* London: University of Virginia Press.

———. (2003). "Witchcraft as the Dark Side of Kinship: Dilemmas of Social Security in New Contexts." *Etnofoor, 16*, 43–61.

Geschiere, P., and Fisiy, C. (1994). "Domesticating Personal Violence: Witchcraft, Courts and Confessions in Cameroon." *Africa: Journal of the International African Institute, 64*(3), 323–41.

Geschiere, P., and Konings, P. (1993). *Itinéraires d'accumulation au Caméroun.* Leiden: Afrika Studie Centrum.

Giddens, A. (1979). *Central Problems in Social Theory.* London: Macmillan.

———. (1991). *Modernity and Self-Identity: Self and Society in the Late Modern Age.* Cambridge: Polity.

Gilligan, C. (1982). *In a Different Voice: Psychological Theory and Women's Development.* Cambridge, MA: Harvard University Press.

Ginsburg, F. D. (1998). *Contested Lives: The Abortion Debate in an American Community.* Berkeley: University of California Press.

Ginsburg, F. D., and Rapp, R. (1991). "The Politics of Reproduction." *Annual Review of Anthropology, 20,* 311–43.

———. (1995). *Conceiving the New World Order: The Global Politics of Reproduction.* Berkeley: University of California Press.

Godelier, M. (1992). Corps, parenté, pouvoir(s) chez les Baruya de Nouvelle-Guinée. *Journal de la Société des Océanistes, 94*(1), 3–24.

Goheen, M. (1993). "Les champs appartiennent aux hommes, les récoltes aux femmes: Accumulation dans la region de Nso." In P. Geschiere and P. Konings (Eds.), *Itinéraires d'accumulation au Cameroun* (pp. 241–72). Paris: Karthala.

———. (1996). *Men Own the Fields, Women Own the Crops: Gender and Power in the Cameroon Grassfields.* Madison: University of Wisconsin Press.

Goody, E. (1984). "Parental Strategies: Calculation or Sentiment? Fostering Practices among West Africans." In H. Medick and D. W. Sabean (Eds.), *Interest and Emotion: Essays on the Study of Family and Kinship* (pp. 9–27). Cambridge: Cambridge University Press.

Gottlieb, A. (2004). *The Afterlife Is Where We Come From: The Culture of Infancy in West Africa.* Chicago: University of Chicago Press.

Greenhalgh, S. (1995). *Situating Fertility: Anthropology and Demographic Inquiry.* Cambridge: Cambridge University Press.

Grotevant, H. D. (2007). "Openness in Adoption: Rethinking 'Family' in the US." In M. C. Inhorn (Ed.), *Reproductive Disruptions: Gender, Technology, and Biopolitics in the New Millennium* (pp. 122–44). New York: Berghahn Books.

Gruenais, M. E. (2001). "Un système de santé en mutation: Le cas du Cameroun." *Bulletin de l'APAD, 21.* apad.revues.org/25.

GTZ. (2009). *Rape and Incest in Cameroon: Final Report.* Yaoundé: GTZ.

Gubry, P., and Wautelet, J.-M. (1993). "Population et processus de développement au Cameroun." In *Intégrer Population et Développement: Chaire Quetelet 1990* (pp. 614–67). Louvain-la-Neuve: Academia-L'Harmattan.

Gupta, A. (2002). "Reliving Childhood? The Temporality of Childhood and Narratives of Reincarnation." *Ethnos: Journal of Anthropology, 67*(1), 33–55.

Guthrie, M. (1953). *The Bantu Languages of Western Equatorial Africa.* London: Oxford University Press.

Guttmacher Institute. (2003). "Although Abortion Is Highly Restricted in Cameroon, It Is Not Uncommon among Young Urban Women." *International Family Planning Perspectives, 29*(1), 2–4.

Guyer, J. I. (1984). *Family and Farm in Southern Cameroon* (vol. 15). Boston: Boston University, African Studies Center.

———. (1986). "Indigenous Currencies and the History of Marriage Payments: A Case Study from Cameroon." *Cahiers d'Études Africaines, 26*(104), 577–610.

———. (1996). "Traditions of Invention in Equatorial Africa." *African Studies Review, 39*(3), 1–28.

———. (2005). Comment on "When the Future Decides: Uncertainty and Intentional Action in Contemporary Cameroon" by Jennifer Johnson-Hanks. *Current Anthropology, 46*(3), 379.

Halliburton, M. (2002). "Rethinking Anthropological Studies of the Body: Manas and Bodham in Kerala." *American Anthropologist, 104*(4), 1123–34.

Hanigsberg, J. E. (1995). "Homologizing Pregnancy and Motherhood: A Consideration of Abortion." *Michigan Law Review, 94*(2), 371–418.

Hardacre, H. (1999). *Marketing the Menacing Fetus in Japan.* Berkeley: University of California Press.

Hardin, G. (1974). "Lifeboat Ethics: The Case against Helping the Poor." *BioScience, 24*(10), 561–68.

Haws, R. A., Mashasi, I., Mrisho, M., Schellenberg, J. A., Darmstadt, G. L., and Winch, P. J. (2010). "These Are Not Good Things for Other People to Know": How Rural Tanzanian Women's Experiences of Pregnancy Loss and Early Neonatal Death May Impact Survey Data Quality." *Social Science and Medicine, 71*(10), 1764–72.

Heinonen, S., and Kirkinen, P. (2000). "Pregnancy Outcome after Previous Stillbirth Resulting from Causes Other Than Maternal Conditions and Fetal Abnormalities." *Birth, 27*(1), 33–37.

Henshaw, S. K., Singh, S., and Haas, T. (1999). "Recent Trends in Abortion Rates Worldwide." *International Family Planning Perspectives, 25*(1), 44–48.

Heriot, M. J. (1996). "Fetal Rights versus the Female Body: Contested Domains." *Medical Anthropology Quarterly, 10*(2), 176–94.

Héritier, F. (1984). "Stérilité, aridité, sécheresse: Quelques invariants de la pensée symbolique." In M. Augé and C. Herzlich (Eds.), *Le sens du mal: Anthropologie, histoire, sociologie de la maladie* (pp. 123–54). Paris: Editions des Archives Contemporaines.

———. (2003). "Une anthropologie symbolique du corps." *Journal des Africanistes, 73*(2), 9–26.

Hewson, B. (2001). "Reproductive Autonomy and the Ethics Of Abortion." *Journal of Medical Ethics, 27,* 10–14.

Holtedahl, L. (1993). "Education, Economics and 'The Good Life': Women in Ngaoundéré, Northern Cameroon." In P. Geschiere and P. Konings (Eds.), *Itinéraires d'accumulation au Cameroun* (pp. 273–300). Paris: Karthala.

Holy, L. (1996). *Anthropological Perspectives on Kinship.* London: Pluto.

Houseman, M. (1988). "Social Structure Is Where the Hearth Is: A "Woman's Place" in Beti Society." *Africa, 58*(1), 51–69.

Hubbard, R. (1994). "The Politics of Fetal-Maternal Conflict." In G. Sen and R. Snow (Eds.), *Power and Decision: The Social Control of Reproduction* (pp. 311–24). Cambridge, MA: Harvard University Press.

Hunt, N. R. (2005). "Fertility's Fires and Empty Wombs in Recent Africanist Writing." *Africa, 75*(3), 421–35.

Hunter, M. (2002). "The Materiality of Everyday Sex: Thinking beyond 'Prostitution.'" *African Studies, 61*(1), 99–120.

Inhorn, M. C. (1994). *Quest for Conception: Gender, Infertility, and Egyptian Medical Traditions.* Philadelphia: University of Pennsylvania Press.

———. (1996). *Infertility and Patriarchy: The Cultural Politics of Gender and Family Life in Egypt.* Philadelphia: University of Philadelphia Press.

———. (2003). *Local Babies, Global Science: Gender, Religion, and In Vitro Fertilization in Egypt.* New York: Routledge.

———. (2012). *The New Arab Man: Emergent Masculinities, Technologies, and Islam in the Middle East.* Princeton, NJ: Princeton University Press.

Inhorn, M. C., and Birenbaum-Carmeli, D. (2008). "Assisted Reproductive Technologies and Culture Change." *Annual Review of Anthropology, 37,* 177–234.

Inhorn, M. C., and Van Balen, F. (2002). *Infertility around the Globe: New Thinking on Childlessness, Gender, and Reproductive Technologies.* Berkeley: University of California Press.

Ivry, T. (2009). "The Ultrasonic Picture Show and the Politics of Threatened Life." *Medical Anthropology Quarterly, 23*(3), 189–211.

Jackson, M. (1998). *Minima Ethnographica: Intersubjectivity and the Anthropological Project.* Chicago: University of Chicago Press.

Jackson, M., and Karp, I. (1990). *Personhood and Agency: The Experience of Self and Other in African Cultures.* Uppsala: Acta Universitatis Upsaliensis.

Jeffery, P., and Jeffery, R. (2010). "Only When the Boat Has Started Sinking: A Maternal Death in Rural North India." *Social Science and Medicine, 71*(10), 1711–18.

Jejeebhoy, S. J. (1995). *Women's Education, Autonomy, and Reproductive Behaviour: Experience from Developing Countries.* Oxford: Clarendon.

Jenkins, G. L., and Inhorn, M. C. (2003). "Reproduction Gone Awry: Medical Anthropological Perspectives." *Social Science and Medicine 56*(9), 1831–36.

Johnson, J. M., Thompson, S. L., and Perry, G. J. (1990). "Juju-Soup: The Witch Herbalist's Solution for Infertility." *African Studies Review, 33*(1), 55–64.

Johnson-Hanks, J. (2002a). "The Lesser Shame: Abortion among Educated Women in Southern Cameroon." *Social Science and Medicine, 55*(8), 1337–49.

———. (2002b). "On the Limits of Life Stages in Ethnography: Toward a Theory of Vital Conjunctures." *American Anthropologist, 104*(3), 865–80.

———. (2005). "When the Future Decides: Uncertainty and Intentional Action in Contemporary Cameroon." *Current Anthropology, 46*(3), 363–86.

———. (2006). *Uncertain Honor: Modern Motherhood in an African Crisis.* Chicago: University of Chicago Press.

———. (2007). "Women on the Market: Marriage, Consumption, and the Internet in Urban Cameroon." *American Ethnologist, 34*(4), 642–58.

Johnson-Hanks, J. A., Bachrach, C. A., Morgan, S. P., and Kohler, H. P. (2011). *Understanding Family Change and Variation: Toward a Theory of Conjunctural Action.* Dordrecht: Springer.

Jones, L. S. (2001). "Hope Deferred: Theological Reflections on Reproductive Loss (Infertility, Stillbirth, Miscarriage)." *Modern Theology, 17*(2), 227–45.

Kamdoum, A. (1994). "Planification sanitaire et ajustement structurel au Cameroun." *Dossiers du CEPED, 29*, 12–35.

Kamtcha, Y. M. M. (2004). *Pluralisme thérapeutique au Cameroun: Contribution à la comprehension des conduits de recours multiples.* Yaoundé: IFORD.

Kandiyoti, D. (1988). "Bargaining with Patriarchy." *Gender and Society, 2*(3), 274–90.

Kaufman, S. R., and Morgan, L. M. (2005). "The Anthropology of the Beginnings and Ends of Life." *Annual Review of Anthropology, 34*, 317–62.

Kielmann, K. (1998). "Barren Ground: Contesting Identities of Infertile Women in Pemba, Tanzania." In M. Lock and P. A. Kaufert (Eds.), *Pragmatic Women and Body Politics* (pp. 127–63). Cambridge: Cambridge University Press.

Kim, N. (1999). "Breaking Free from Patriarchy: A Comparative Study of Sex Selection Abortions in Korea and the United States." *UCLA Pacific Basin Law Journal, 17*, 301–26.

Kirmayer, L. J. (1992). "The Body's Insistence on Meaning: Metaphor as Presentation and Representation in Illness Experience." *Medical Anthropology Quarterly, 6*(4), 323–46.

Klaus, M. H., and Kennel, J. (Eds.). (1976). *Maternal-Infant Bonding.* St. Louis: Mosby.

Kleiner-Bossaller, A. (1993). "Kwantacce, the Sleeping Pregnancy, a Hausa Concept." In G. Ludwar-Ene and M. Reh (Eds.), *Focus on Women in Africa* (pp. 17–29). Bayreuth: African Studies Series.

Konings, P. (1995). "Plantation Labour and Economic Crisis in Cameroon." *Development and Change, 26,* 525–49.

Koster, W. (2003). *Secret Strategies: Women and Abortion in Yoruba Society, Nigeria.* Amsterdam: Aksant.

———. (2010). "Linking Two Opposites of Pregnancy Loss: Induced Abortion and Infertility in Yoruba Society, Nigeria." *Social Science and Medicine, 71*(10), 1788–95.

Krumeich, J. S. M. (1994). *The Blessings of Motherhood: Health, Pregnancy and Child Care in Dominica.* Amsterdam: Het Spinhuis.

Laburthe-Tolra, P. (1981). *Minlaaba: Les seigneurs de la forêt.* Paris: Karthala.

———. (1985). *Initiations et sociétés secrètes au Cameroun: Les mystères de la nuit.* Paris: Karthala.

Lambert, H., and McDonald, M. (Eds.). (2009). *Social Bodies.* New York: Berghahn Books.

Lantum, D. N. (1985). "The Sterility Problem in Cameroon (a Socio-Demographic Aspect)." In D. N. Lantum (Ed.), *The Sterility Phenomenon in Cameroon in 1985: Report of CUSS-Yaounde, 29 July–3rd August 1985.* Yaoundé: UCHS/CUSS Occasional Paper No. 2.

Larsen, U. (1995). "Differentials in Infertility in Cameroon and Nigeria." *Population Studies, 49*(2), 329–46.

Layne, L. L. (1997). "Breaking the Silence: An Agenda for a Feminist Discourse of Pregnancy Loss." *Feminist Studies, 23*(2), 289–316.

———. (2003). *Motherhood Lost: A Feminist Account of Pregnancy Loss in America.* New York: Routledge.

———. (2006). "A Women's Health Model for Pregnancy Loss: A Call for a New Standard of Care." *Feminist Studies, 32*(3), 573–600.

Leclerc-Madlala, S. (2003). "Transactional Sex and the Pursuit of Modernity." *Social Dynamics: A Journal of African Studies, 29*(2), 213–33.

Lee, B. S. (1992). "The Influence of Rural-Urban Migration on Migrant's Fertility Behavior in Cameroon." *International Migration Review, 26*(4), 1416–47.

Leh, J. G. (1987). *Les soins de santé primaires dans les pays du tiers monde:* À propos d'*une expérience personnelle chez les Banen du Cameroun de 1981 à 1984.* Yaoundé: Université de Yaoundé I.

Leonard, L. (2002). "'Looking for Children': The Search for Fertility among the Sara of Southern Chad." *Medical Anthropology Quarterly, 21*(1), 79–112.

Letherby, G. (1993). "The Meanings of Miscarriage." *Women's Studies International Forum, 16*(2), 165–80.

———. (1999). "Other Than Mother and Mothers as Others: The Experience of Motherhood and Non-motherhood in Relation to 'Infertility' and 'Involuntary Childlessness.'" *Women's Studies International Forum, 22*(3), 359–72.

Liboko Ndabanga, S. L. (2001). *Facteurs explicatifs des comportements sexuels des femmes en Afrique Subsaharienne: Cas du Cameroun.* Yaoundé: IFORD.

LiPuma, E. (1998). "Modernity and Forms of Personhood in Melanesia." In M. Lambek and A. Strathern (Eds.), *Bodies and Persons: Comparative Perspectives from Africa and Melanesia* (pp. 53–79). Cambridge: Cambridge University Press.

Littlewood, J. (1999). "From the Invisibility of Miscarriage to an Attribution of Life." *Anthropology and Medicine, 6*(2), 217–30.

Lloyd, C. B., and Mensch, B. S. (2008). "Marriage and Childbirth as Factors in Dropping Out from School: An Analysis of DHS Data from Sub-Saharan Africa." *Population Studies: A Journal of Demography, 62*(1), 1–13.

Lock, M. (1993a). "Cultivating the Body: Anthropology and Epistemologies of Bodily Practice and Knowledge." *Annual Review of Anthropology, 22*, 133–55.

———. (1993b). *Encounters with Aging: Mythologies of Menopause in Japan and North America.* Berkeley: University of California Press.

Lock, M., and Kaufert, P. A. (1997). *Pragmatic Women and Body Politics.* New York: Cambridge University Press.

Lyon, M. L. (1997). "The Material Body, Social Processes and Emotion: 'Techniques of the Body' Revisited." *Body and Society, 3*(1), 83–101.

Mackenzie, C., and Stoljar, N. (2000). *Relational Autonomy: Feminist Perspectives on Autonomy, Agency, and the Social Self.* New York: Oxford University Press.

Macklon, N. S., Geraedts, J. P. M., and Fauser, B. C. J. M. (2002). "Conception to Ongoing Pregnancy: The "Black Box" of Early Pregnancy Loss." *Human Reproduction Update, 8*(4), 333–43.

Mahoney, M. (1994). "Victimization or Oppression? Women's Lives, Violence and Agency." In M. A. Fineman and R. Mykitiuk (Eds.), *The Public Nature of Private Violence* (pp. 59–92). New York: Routledge.

Mallart Guimera, L. (1981). *Ni dos ni ventre: Religion, magie et sorcellerie Evuzok.* Paris: Société d'Ethnographie.

Margolis, M. L. (1993). "Review: Death without Weeping." *American Anthropologist, 95*(2), 495–97.

Mauss, M. (1950). "Les techniques du corps." In M. Mauss (Ed.), *Sociologie et anthropologie* (pp. 363–86). Paris: PUF.

Maynard, K. (2004). *Making Kedjom Medicine: A History of Public Health and Well-Being in Cameroon.* Westport: Praeger.

Médard, J. F. (2001). "Décentralisation du système de santé publique et ressources humaines au Cameroun." *Bulletin de l'APAD, 21. apad.revues.org/document35.html.*

Meekers, D., and Calvès, A. E. (1997). "'Main' Girlfriends, Girlfriends, Marriage, and Money: The Social Context of HIV Risk Behaviour in Sub-Saharan Africa." *Health Transition Review, 7*, 361–75.

Mengue, A. (1982). *L'Est Camerounais: Une géographie du sous-peuplement et de la marginalité.* Bordeaux: Université de Bordeaux.

Meyers, D. T. (2001). "The Rush to Motherhood: Pronatalist Discourse and Women's Autonomy." *Signs, 26*, 735–74.

Ministère de la Santé Publique Cameroun. (1993a). *National Declaration on the Implementation of the Reorientation of Primary Health Care.* Yaoundé: Ministère de la Santé Publique Cameroun.

———. (1993b). *Alimentation des enfants de 0 à 5 ans, femmes enceintes et allaitantes dans les provinces de l'Extreme Nord, Est, Ouest et dans la ville de Douala (revue de la literature).* Yaoundé: Ministère de la Santé Publique Cameroun.

———. (1994). *Rapport de l'étude ethnographique dans la province de l'Est.*

———. (1995). *Identification des problèmes nutritionnels des enfants de 0 à 5 ans, femmes enceintes et allaitantes à partir des données de la phase d'exploration.* Yaoundé: Ministère de la Santé Publique Cameroun.

———. (2001a). *Declaration of the National Population Policy.* Yaoundé: Ministère de la Santé Publique.

———. (2001b). *Politique et normes des services de la santé de la reproduction.* Yaoundé: Ministère de la Santé Publique.

———. (2009). *Stratégie sectorielle de santé 2001–2015.* Yaoundé: Ministère de la Santé Publique.

———. (2011). *Plan nationale de développement sanitaire (PNDS) 2011–2015.* Yaoundé: Ministère de la Santé Publique.

———. (n.d.). *Module sur le recouvrement des couts: Draft no. 1.* Yaoundé: Ministère de la Santé Publique.

Mitchell, L. M. (2004). "Women's Experiences of Unexpected Ultrasound Findings." *Journal of Midwifery and Women's Health, 49*(3), 228–34.

————. (2006). "Body and Illness: Considering Visayan Filipino Children's Perspectives within Local and Global Relationships of Inequality." *Medical Anthropology, 25*(4), 331–73.

Molel Belika, L. (2008). *La notion de la personne chez les Banen du Cameroun.* Yaoundé: Université de Yaoundé I.

Monach, J. H. (1993). *Childless, No Choice: The Experience of Involuntary Childlessness.* New York: Routledge.

Morgan, L. M. (1996). "Fetal Relationality in Feminist Philosophy: An Anthropological Critique." *Hypatia, 11*(3), 47–70.

Moupou, M., and Akei Mbanga, L. (2008). "Désengagement de l'État et réponses paysannes au Cameroun." *Les Cahiers d'Outre-Mer, 61*(241), 163–83.

Nahar, P. (2007). *Childless in Bangladesh: Suffering and Resilience among Rural and Urban Women.* Amsterdam: University of Amsterdam.

Nahar, P., Sharma, A., Sabin, K., Begum, L., Ahsan, S. K., and Baqui, A. H. (2000). "Living with Infertility: Experiences among Urban Slum Populations in Bangladesh." *Reproductive Health Matters, 8*(15), 33–44.

Nasah, B. T. (1978). "Aetiology of Infertility in the Came Roune." *Nigerian Medical Journal, 8*(5), 452–56.

Nations, M. K., Misago, C., Fonseca, W., Correia, L. L., and Campbell, O. M. R. (1997). "Women's Hidden Transcripts about Abortion in Brazil." *Social Science and Medicine, 44*(12), 1833–45.

Nelson, H. D., Dobert, M., McDonald, G. C., McLaughlin, J., Marvin, B., and Moeller, P. W. (1974). *Area Handbook for the United Republic of Cameroon.* Washington, DC: Foreign Area Studies.

Newman, L. F. (1985). *Women's Medicine: A Cross-Cultural Study of Indigenous Fertility Regulation.* New Brunswick, NJ: Rutgers University Press.

Ngo Baleba, A. (2003). *Ils ont construit l'Église de l'Est Cameroun 1900–2000: Des Pères spiritains se racontent.* Czestochowa: Educator.

Ngo Bell, V. R. (1990). *Les familles Camerounaises face au planning familiale: Intégration ou rejet?* Yaoundé: Université de Yaoundé I.

Ngono, M. G. (2005). *Facteurs de la pratique de la prévention antivectorielle dans les ménages de l'Est Cameroun.* Yaoundé: Université de Yaoundé I.

Nguyen, T. H. (2011). *Rape Experiences and the Limits of Women's Agency in Contemporary Post-reform Vietnam.* Amsterdam: University of Amsterdam.

Nichter, M. (1981). "Idioms of Distress: Alternatives in the Expression of Psychosocial Distress; A Case Study from South India." *Culture, Medicine and Psychiatry, 5*(4), 379–408.

Niger-Thomas, M. (2000). "Buying Futures: The Upsurge of Female Entrepreneurship; Crossing the Formal and Informal Divide in Southwest Cameroon." PhD diss., Leiden University.

Njikam Savage, O. M. (1992). "Artificial Donor Insemination in Yaoundé: Some Socio-cultural Considerations." *Social Science and Medicine, 35,* 297–306.

———. (1996). "'Children of the Rope' and Other Aspects of Pregnancy Loss in Cameroon." In R. Cecil (Ed.), *The Anthropology of Pregnancy Loss: Comparative Studies in Miscarriage, Stillbirth, and Neonatal Death* (pp. 95–107). Oxford: Berg.

———. (1998). "Adolescents' Beliefs and Perceptions towards Sexuality in Urban Cameroon." In B. Kuate-Defo (Ed.), *Sexuality and Reproductive Health during Adolescence in Africa, with Special Reference to Cameroon* (pp. 77–90). Ottawa: University of Ottawa Press.

Nkwi, P. (1985). "Traditional Female Militancy in a Modern Context." In J.-C. Barbier (Ed.), *Femmes du Cameroun: Mères pacifiques, femmes rebelles* (pp. 181–91). Paris: Karthala.

Notermans, C. (1999). *Verhalen in veelvoud: Vrouwen in Kameroen over polygynie en christendom.* Nijmegen: Valkhof Pers.

———. (2003). "Nomads in Kinship: Fosterage and the Self in Cameroon." *Focaal* (42), 89–104.

———. (2008). "The Emotional World of Kinship: Children's Experiences of Fosterage in East Cameroon." *Childhood: A Global Journal of Child Research, 15*(3), 355–77.

Nseke, M. M. (2002). *La planification familiale au Cameroun: Les facteurs limitants.* Yaoundé: Université de Yaoundé I.

Nsoa Mbondo, P. (2008). *Besoins non satisfaits en matière d'éducation sur les complications obstétricales au Cameroun: Niveaux et déterminants.* Yaoundé: IFORD.

Nyamnjoh, F. B. (2002). "'A Child Is One Person's Only in the Womb': Domestication, Agency and Subjectivity in the Cameroonian Grassfields." In R. Werbner (Ed.), *Postcolonial Subjectivities in Africa* (pp. 111–38). London: Zed Books.

———. (2005). "Fishing in Troubled Waters: Disquettes and Thiofs in Dakar." *Africa, 75*(3), 295–324.

Nyobia, A. (2006). "Avortement clandestin: Le business 'fertile.'" *Cameroon-Tribune,* June 29. *www.cameroon-tribune.cm*

O'Brien, P. K. (2000). "The Reconstruction, Rehabilitation and Reconfiguration of the British Industrial Revolution as a Conjuncture in Global History." *Itinerario, 3*(4), 117–34.

Olarte Sierra, M. F. (2010). *Achieving the Desirable Nation: Abortion and Antenatal Testing in Colombia; The Case of Amniocentesis.* Amsterdam: University of Amsterdam.

Olivier de Sardan, J. P., Moumouni, A., and Souley, A. (2000). "'L'accouchement c'est la guerre': Accoucher en milieu rural nigérien." *Afrique Contemporaine, 195,* 136–54.

Ombolo, J. P. (1991). *Sexe et société en Afrique noire: L'anthropologie sexuelle Beti; Essai analytique, critique et comparatif.* Paris: L'Harmattan.

O'Neill, J. (1985). *Five Bodies: The Human Shape of Modern Society.* Ithaca, NY: Cornell University Press.

Ortner, S. B. (2006). *Anthropology and Social Theory: Culture, Power, and the Acting Subject.* Durham, NC: Duke University Press.

Owono Essomba, R., Bryant, M., and Bodart, C. (1993). "The Reorientation of Primary Health Care in Cameroon: Rationale, Obstacles and Constraints." *Health Policy and Planning, 8*(3), 232–39.

Oyono, F. (1967). *The Old Man and the Medal.* London: Heinemann.

Patel, T. (2007). *Sex-Selective Abortion in India: Gender, Society, and New Reproductive Technologies.* London: Sage.

Paxson, H. (2004). *Making Modern Mothers: Ethics and Family Planning in Urban Greece.* Berkeley: University of California Press.

Petchesky, R. P. (1980). Reproductive Freedom: Beyond "a Woman's Right to Choose." *Signs, 5*(4), 661–85.

———. (1987). "Fetal Images: The Power of Visual Culture in the Politics of Reproduction." *Feminist Studies, 13*(2), 263–92.

Piot, C. D. (1999). *Remotely Global: Village Modernity in West Africa.* Chicago: University of Chicago Press.

Pollack, S. (2000). "Reconceptualizing Women's Agency and Empowerment." *Women and Criminal Justice, 12*(1), 75–89.

Pool, R. (2003). *Dialogue and the Interpretation of Illness: Conversations in a Cameroon Village.* Amsterdam: Het Spinhuis.

Poulin, M. (2007). "Sex, Money, and Premarital Partnerships in Southern Malawi." *Social Science and Medicine, 65*(11), 2383–93.

Radcliffe-Brown, A. R. (1940). "On Joking Relationships." *Africa: Journal of the International African Institute, 13*(3), 195–210.

Rahman, A., Katzive, L., and Henshaw, S. K. (1998). "A Global Review of Laws on Induced Abortion, 1985–1997." *International Family Planning Perspectives, 24*(2), 56–64.

Rai, R., and Regan, L. (2006). Recurrent Miscarriage. *Lancet, 368*(9535), 601–10.

Rapp, R. (2000). *Testing Women, Testing the Fetus: The Social Impact of Amniocentesis in America*. New York: Routledge.

Regan, L., and Rai, R. (2000). "Epidemiology and the Medical Causes of Miscarriage." *Best Practice and Research Clinical Obstetrics and Gynaecology, 14*(5), 839–54.

Renne, E. P. (1996). "The Pregnancy That Doesn't Stay: The Practice and Perception of Abortion by Ekiti Yoruba Women." *Social Science and Medicine, 42*(4), 483–94.

———. (2003). "Changing Assessments of Abortion in a Northern Nigerian Town." In A. M. Basu (Ed.), *The Sociocultural and Political Aspects of Abortion: Global Perspectives* (pp. 119–38). Westport, CT: Praeger.

———. (2006). "Abortion as Illegal Conduct and Its Sequelae in Nigeria." *Curare, 29*(1), 81–96.

Retel-Laurentin, A. (1974). *Infécondité en Afrique noire: Maladies et conséquences sociales*. Paris: Masson.

Rice, P. L. (2000). "When the Baby Falls! The Cultural Construction of Miscarriage among Hmong Women in Australia." *Women and Health, 30*(1), 85–103.

Richards, S. C. (2002). "'Spoiling the Womb': Definitions, Aetiologies and Responses to Infertility in North West Province, Cameroon." *African Journal of Reproductive Health, 6*(1), 84–94.

Romaniuk, A. (1961). *L'aspect démographique de la stérilité des femmes Congolaises*. Leopoldville: Editions de l'université.

———. (1968). "Infertility in Tropical Africa." In J. C. Caldwell and C. Okonjo (Eds.), *The Population of Tropical Africa* (pp. 214–24). London: Longmans.

Rosenthal, G. (2003). "The Healing Effects of Storytelling: On the Conditions of Curative Storytelling in the Context of Research and Counseling." *Qualitative Inquiry, 9*(6), 915–33.

———. (2004). "Biographical Research." In C. Seale, G. Gobo, J. F. Gubrium, and D. Silverman (Eds.), *Qualitative Research Practice* (pp. 48–64). New York: Sage.

———. (2006). "The Narrated Life Story: In the Interrelation between Experience, Memory and Narration." In K. Milnes, C. Horrocks, N. Kelly, B. Roberts, and D. Robinson (Eds.), *Narrative, Memory, Knowledge: Representations, Aesthetics, Contexts* (pp. 1–16). Huddersfield: University of Huddersfield Press.

Ruddick, S. (1980). "Maternal Thinking." *Feminist Studies, 6*(2), 342–67.

Rylko-Bauer, B. (1996). "Abortion from a Crosscultural Perspective: An Introduction." *Social Science and Medicine, 42*(4), 479–82.

Sahlins, M. (1985). *Islands of History*. Chicago: University of Chicago Press.

Sala-Diakanda, D. (2000). "La positions des gouvernements Africains vis-à-vis des politiques démographiques en matière de fécondité." In P. Vimard, B. C. Zanou, and M. E. Z. de Cosio (Eds.), *Politiques démographiques et transition de la fécondité en Afrique* (pp. 13–45). Paris: L'Harmattan.

Sandelowski, M., and Jones, L. C. (1996). "'Healing Fictions': Stories of Choosing in the Aftermath of the Detection of Fetal Anomalies." *Social Science and Medicine, 42*(3), 353–61.

Sargent, C. F. (1982). *The Cultural Context of Therapeutic Choice: Obstetrical Care Decisions among the Bariba of Benin*. Dordrecht: D. Reidel.

———. (1989). *Maternity, Medicine, and Power: Reproductive Decisions in Urban Benin*. Berkeley: University of California Press.

Scheper-Hughes, N. (1992). *Death without Weeping: The Violence of Everyday Life in Brazil*. Berkeley: University of California Press.

Scheper-Hughes, N., and Lock, M. M. (1987). "The Mindful Body: A Prolegomenon to Future Work in Medical Anthropology." *Medical Anthropology Quarterly, 1*(1), 6–41.

Schneider, E. M. (1993). "Feminism and the False Dichotomy of Victimization and Agency." *New York Law School Law Review, 38*, 387–99.

Schuster, S. (2005). "Abortion in the Moral World of the Cameroon Grassfields." *Reproductive Health Matters, 26*, 130–38.

———. (2010). "Women's Experiences of the Abortion Law in Cameroon: 'What Really Matters.'" *Reproductive Health Matters, 18*(35), 137–44.

Scott, J. C. (1990). *Domination and the Arts of Resistance: Hidden Transcripts*. New Haven, CT: Yale University Press.

Sharma, P. P., Salihu, H. M., and Kirby, R. S. (2007). "Stillbirth Recurrence in a Population of Relatively Low-Risk Mothers." *Paediatric and Perinatal Epidemiology, 21*(s1), 24–30.

Simpson, B. (2007). "Negotiating the Therapeutic Gap: Prenatal Diagnostics and Termination of Pregnancy in Sri Lanka." *Bioethical Inquiry, 4*(3), 207–15.

Sobo, E. J. (1993). *One Blood: The Jamaican Body*. New York: State University of New York Press.

Sökefeld, M. (1999). "Debating Self, Identity, and Culture in Anthropology." *Current Anthropology, 40*(4), 417–48.

Sous-préfecture de Bélabo. (2007). *Procès-verbal de passation de commandement entre mm. Engamba Emmanuel Ledoux, sous-préfet sortant, et Embe David, sous-préfet entrant de l'arrondissement de Bélabo*. Bélabo: Sous-préfecture de Bélabo.

Spiro, M. E. (1993). "Is the Western Conception of the Self 'Peculiar' within the Context of the World Cultures?" *Ethos, 21*(2), 107–53.

Stasch, R. (2009). *Society of Others: Kinship and Mourning in a West Papuan Place.* Berkeley: University of California Press.

Strathern, M. (1995). *The Relation: Issues in Complexity and Scale.* Cambridge: Prickly Pear Press.

Sundby, J., Mboge, R., and Sonko, S. (1998). "Infertility in the Gambia: Frequency and Health Care Seeking." *Social Science and Medicine, 46*(7), 891–99.

Svanemyr, J., and Sundby, J. (2007). "The Social Context of Induced Abortions among Young Couples in Cote d'Ivoire." *African Journal of Reproductive Health, 11*(2), 13–23.

Tantchou, J., and Wilson, E. (2000). *Post-Cairo Reproductive Health Policies and Programs: A Study of Five Francophone African Countries* (vol. 6). Washington, DC: The POLICY Project.

Tawfik, L., and Watkins, S. C. (2007). "Sex in Geneva, Sex in Lilongwe, and Sex in Balaka." *Social Science and Medicine, 64*(5), 1090–101.

Taylor, C. C. (1992). *Milk, Honey, and Money: Changing Concepts in Rwandan Healing.* Washington, DC: Smithsonian Institution Press.

Thomson, J. J. (1971). "A Defense of Abortion." *Philosophy and Public Affairs, 1*(1), 47–66.

Thompson, C. (2005). *Making Parents: The Ontological Choreography of Reproductive Technologies.* Cambridge: MIT Press.

Tsala Tsala, J. P. (1996). "Grossesse et interdits chez les Beti." *Cahiers de Sociologie Économique et Culturelle, 25,* 85–94.

Turner, T. (1995). "Social Body and Embodied Subject: Bodiliness, Subjectivity, and Sociality among the Kayapo." *Cultural Anthropology, 10*(2), 143–70.

UN CEDAW (Committee on the Elimination of Discrimination against Women). (1999). *Consideration of Reports Submitted by States Parties under Article 18 of the Convention on the Elimination of All Forms of Discrimination against Women: Cameroon.* Geneva: United Nations.

UN CRC. (2000). *Committee on the Rights of the Child: Consideration of Reports Submitted by States Parties under Article 44 of the Convention; Cameroon.* Geneva: United Nations.

Utas, M. (2005). "Victimcy, Girlfriending, Soldiering: Tactic Agency in a Young Woman's Social Navigation in the Liberian War Zone." *Anthropological Quarterly, 78*(2), 403–30.

van Beek, W. E. A. (1994). "The Innocent Sorcerer: Coping with Evil in Two African Societies (Kapsiki and Dogon)." In T. D. Blakely, W. E. A. v. Beek, and D. L. Thomson (Eds.), *Religion in Africa: Experience and Expression* (pp. 196–228). London: James Currey.

van der Geest, S. (1982a). "The Efficiency of Inefficiency: Medicine Distribution in South Cameroon." *Social Science and Medicine, 16*(24), 2145–53.

———. (1982b). "The Secondary Importance of Primary Health Care in South Cameroon." *Culture, Medicine and Psychiatry, 6,* 365–83.

van der Sijpt, E. (2007). "Marginal Motherhood: The Ambiguous Experience of Pregnancy-Loss in Cameroon." *Medische Antropologie: Tijdschrift over gezondheid en cultuur, 19*(2), 245–68.

———. (2010). "'Filling with Force': Reproductive Loss Reconsidered." *Viennese Ethnomedicine Newsletter, 12*(2–3), 21–27.

———. (2013). "Focusing on Force and Forms: Reproductive Loss Reconsidered." In S. Earle, C. Komaromy, and L. Layne (Eds.), *Understanding Reproductive Loss: International Perspectives on Life, Death, and Fertility* (pp. 105–16). Surrey: Ashgate.

van der Sijpt, E., and Notermans, C. (2010). "Perils to Pregnancies: On Social Sorrows and Strategies Surrounding Pregnancy Loss in Cameroon." *Medical Anthropology Quarterly, 24*(3), 381–98.

van de Walle, E., and Renne, E. P. (2001). *Regulating Menstruation: Beliefs, Practices, Interpretations.* Chicago: University of Chicago Press.

Van Hollen, C. C. (2003). *Birth on the Threshold: Childbirth and Modernity in South India.* Berkeley: University of California Press.

van Santen, J. (1993). "Dot, commerce et contrebande: Stratégies d'accumulation chez les femmes 'islamisées' de Mokolo." In P. Geschiere and P. Konings (Eds.), *Itinéraires d'accumulation au Cameroun* (pp. 301–34). Paris: Karthala.

Velghe-Scherpereel, G., and van de Wouwer-Leunda, P. (1996). *Profil femmes et développement au Cameroun.* Yaoundé: Ambassade Royale des Pays-Bas.

Verhoef, H. (2005). "A Child Has Many Mothers." *Childhood, 12*(3), 369–90.

Vigh, H. (2006). *Navigating Terrains of War: Youth and Soldiering in Guinea-Bissau.* New York: Berghahn Books.

———. (2009). "Motion Squared: A Second Look at the Concept of Social Navigation." *Anthropological Theory, 9*(4), 419–38.

Vincent, J.-F. (1976). *Traditions et transition: Entretiens avec des femmes Beti du Sud-Cameroun; Mariage et situation pré-coloniale, anciens rites de femmes, magie et sorcellerie, réactions à la christianisation.* Paris: ORSTOM.

———. (2001). *Femmes Beti entre deux mondes: Entretiens dans la forêt du Cameroun.* Paris: Karthala.

Wagner-Pacifici, R. (2004). *Theorizing the Standoff: Contingency in Action.* Cambridge: Cambridge University Press.

Wakam, J. (1994). *De la pertinence des théories "économistes" de fécondité dans le contexte socio-culturel camerounais et negro-africain*. Yaoundé: IFORD.

Wankah, C., Ndongo, N., and Abega, M. (1998). "Synthèse du rapport sur l'étude de cas de l'IB/REOSSP au Cameroun." In Ministère de la Santé Publique Cameroun (Ed.), *La mise en oeuvre de la réorientation des soins de santé primaires au Cameroun*. Yaoundé: Ministère de la Santé Publique.

Whittaker, A. (2002). "'The Truth of Our Day by Day Lives': Abortion Decision Making in Rural Thailand." *Culture, Health and Sexuality, 4*(1), 1–20.

———. (2004). *Abortion, Sin, and the State in Thailand*. New York: Routledge.

———. (2010). *Abortion in Asia: Local Dilemmas, Global Politics*. New York: Berghahn Books.

Whyte, S. R. (1997). *Questioning Misfortune: The Pragmatics of Uncertainty in Eastern Uganda*. Cambridge: Cambridge University Press.

———. (2002). "Subjectivity and Subjunctivity: Hoping for Health in Eastern Uganda." In R. Werbner (Ed.), *Postcolonial Subjectivities in Africa* (pp. 171–90). London: Zed.

World Health Organization. (2007). *Maternal Mortality in 2005: Estimates Developed by WHO, UNICEF, UNFPA and the World Bank*. Geneva: WHO.

Wynn, F. (2002). "The Early Relationship of Mother and Pre-infant: Merleau-Ponty and Pregnancy." *Nursing Philosophy, 3*(1), 4–14.

Yana, S. D. (1995). *A la recherché des modèles culturels de la fécondité au Cameroun: Une étude exploratoire aupres de Bamiléké et Beti de la ville et de la campagne*. Yaoundé: IFORD.

Zaman, S., and Chowdury, A. M. R. (1998). "Exploring Women's Perception of Reproduction through Body Mapping: A Research Note from Bangladesh." *Medische Antropologie: Tijdschrift over gezondheid en cultuur, 10*(1), 69–75.

Index

www.ingramcontent.com/pod-product-compliance
Lightning Source LLC
Chambersburg PA
CBHW030644270326
41929CB00007B/206